THE 10-HOUR DIET

THE 10-HOUR DIET

The Ultimate Guide to
Time-Restricted Eating

Jeannette Hyde

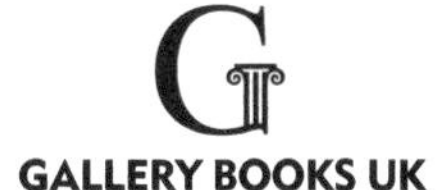

GALLERY BOOKS UK

G

First published in Great Britain by Gallery Books,
an imprint of Simon & Schuster UK Ltd, 2021

3 5 7 9 10 8 6 4 2

Simon & Schuster UK Ltd
1st Floor
222 Gray's Inn Road
London WC1X 8HB

www.simonandschuster.co.uk
www.simonandschuster.com.au
www.simonandschuster.co.in

Simon & Schuster Australia, Sydney
Simon & Schuster India, New Delhi

A CIP catalogue record for this book
is available from the British Library

Paperback ISBN: 978-1-3985-0269-7
eBook ISBN: 978-1-3985-0270-3

Typeset in Stone Serif by M Rules
Printed in the UK by CPI Group (UK) Ltd, Croydon, CR0 4YY

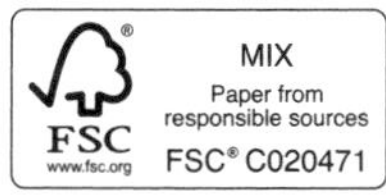

To Markus, Max and Hanna

IMPORTANT NOTE

This book is concerned with diet and well-being and does not give medical advice. You should not alter your dietary patterns without seeking medical advice if you are on medication, undergoing medical treatment, pregnant or have a pre-existing physical or psychological condition that may make you vulnerable. Your diet is your choice and your responsibility. If you have any doubts or concerns you should consult your GP or other appropriately qualified professional adviser.

CONTENTS

THE 10-HOUR DIET

AUTHOR'S NOTE

As the nation tries to arrest the Covid-19 virus with more lockdowns, is it frivolous to launch a new diet book? For some people, the lack of structure at the beginning of the virus outbreak, and sudden confinement at home, made managing their weight more difficult. As many as a third of us put on weight during the first 2020 lockdown. But could this new life – commuting and socialising less, and working from home more – if viewed from a new angle, present one of the best opportunities in decades to get healthy by taking control of the times we eat, which we now know are vital to our weight and health?

Researchers have established that *when* we eat can have a powerfully positive influence on our weight, blood sugar balance, heart and immune system. Maybe now is the perfect opportunity to easily implement a new routine? Now that we don't have to pack onto commuter trains at dawn, cheek by jowl, or go to those early-evening-wine networking soirées, could we nudge breakfast back a bit later and bring supper and that glass of wine forward? In our lunch break, could we get a head start on tonight's meal and do some dinner prep? At weekends, will breakfast or lunch become the new supper, now that pubs and restaurants have to shut early?

Pundits predict office working will never be the same following the Covid-19 pandemic. They say we'll never go back to working five days a week in an office, getting up at the crack of dawn, having an exhausting commute and arriving home late. Maybe this is going to provide a chance to eat earlier, which could have a massive impact on the health of the nation.

Over the past few years, I have been following the emerging research on time-restricted eating (TRE) and have tried many different combinations of eating times with hundreds of clients in my group workshops, one-to-one nutritional therapy sessions in London and on my 'Reboot. Nourish. Empower' retreats in Spain. What I have learnt is that the sweet spot to get the health benefits from TRE is to eat in a 10-hour time slot, finishing between 6pm and 8pm at the latest.

What I have also learnt is that the devil is in the detail with TRE. And that is why I have written this book, which combines what we are learning from the very latest studies with my own experience in clinical practice. The internet is full of conflicting advice on TRE, which is a form of intermittent fasting. This book is designed to help you overcome the difficulties and areas of confusion so you can follow new eating times with successful results – and learn what can and cannot be consumed during the fast. I answer many of your questions and uncertainties so you can reap the benefits.

Before becoming a nutritional therapist, I was a senior

editor of a national newspaper. I used to get up when it was still dark, do a long commute eating a croissant and coffee on the train, snack at my desk on and off throughout the day, go home in the dark and drink half a bottle of wine when I got there. One morning, I woke up and couldn't move my neck or spine. Burnout presents itself in many different forms and this was how it affected me. It was as if I physically had been in a car crash. I was waking up crying every day. My body and mind just said: 'No more.' I left my beloved writing profession and spent a year at home getting well – cooking from scratch, walking in daylight again and reconnecting with my young family.

I then enrolled on a four-year BSc degree at the University of Westminster to become a nutritional therapist. As a journalist, I'd had to have an enquiring mind. I wanted to learn about managing health through diet and lifestyle. I had learnt first-hand what happens when these aren't right, so I wanted to be able to critique and interpret scientific literature for myself and to share it with others beyond the low-fat and calorie-counting practices of the time.

Although I wouldn't ever want to go through a burnout again, I am grateful for where it led me. In 2015, I wrote *The Gut Makeover*, which jumped on new science regarding the microbiome and was at the forefront of the gut-health revolution, which continues to this day. I now combine writing, research, and clinical practice and group work, to reach as many people as possible. I have worked with a wide range of individuals, from those on benefits to billionaires. Guiding people on their health journeys and providing support to everyone I meet, to help them be healthy and strong, is my passion.

I have written this book to share the latest research on time-restricted eating and to help make it work for you.

Jeannette Hyde,
BSc (Hons) Nutritional Therapy, mBANT, CNHC

CHAPTER ONE

The Simple Science of Eating in a 10-Hour Time Slot Each Day

This is not the first diet book that has been published. Nor is the 10-hour Diet the first weight solution offered. But there is still a reason why you're reading this book.

Dieting is a relatively new phenomenon. At no other time in human history has there been such a preoccupation with losing weight. And many of the ways in which we try to do it are new too: counting calories; expensive gym membership; foods with natural fats sucked out and replaced with artificial sugars to make them palatable. But still, the diet industry continues to grow.

So, maybe the counting-calories thing and doing-more-exercise approach isn't working. Maybe we don't have to count calories every day to lose weight. If no other society in history has done it, perhaps the solution is even simpler.

Think about it.

Our ancestors used to structure their days very differently

to us: rising with the sun, eating during the day and sleeping when darkness fell. As a result of our modern living patterns, not only have the foods we eat changed, but timings for eating have too. Here I'll explain a new, natural, kinder approach to health and weight loss which will help you feel younger and lose weight and simultaneously support heart health and help protect you from developing type 2 diabetes.

Let me introduce you to the 10-Hour Diet. It is in the family of intermittent fasting diets and is based on time-restricted eating (TRE). This means simply eating your meals in a 10-hour time slot each day, in tune with your body's natural rhythms, and not eating for the other 14 hours.

Time-restricted eating has a track record of proven results. Now, there is even more scientific research to back it up, which means we can refine our approach. I have worked with hundreds of clients in my nutritional practice on Harley Street, all to varying degrees of success, and in this book I will share what the research shows: a newer, easier form of intermittent fasting which can be implemented with comfort for the long term. You simply eat your existing diet within only 10 hours of the day. This enables your body to have a long overnight fast of 14 hours, most of which you'll be sleeping through anyway. These 14 hours without food are when your body turns its attention to burning fat and remodelling almost every organ in your body to help you stay young and healthy for longer.

The human body is a fantastic piece of machinery that doesn't just grind to a halt if 2,000 calories haven't been poured into it one day. It has mechanisms that get switched on to help us survive and power up many organs in the body to operate when food is scarce, the research of which I will walk you through here and in Chapter 2.

We come from hunter-gatherers who had naturally enforced periods of feast and famine led by daylight (when we could hunt) and darkness (which forced us to sleep).

Let's dive here into time-restricted eating (TRE), originally termed time-restricted feeding (TRF), and why eating in a 10-hour slot could help us all reset.

Between 2012 and 2015, a group of scientists at the Salk Institute in San Diego published studies which were revolutionary and would change the landscape of intermittent fasting forever.

They took mice and divvied them up into groups and fed them all exactly the same daily calorie counts of various chow concoctions, high in fat and sugar. They conducted a series of studies for periods of time between four weeks and four months. The only aspect that was different between the groups was the timing of when the mice could eat said chow.

The studies found that the mice who could only eat their food in eight and nine-hour blocks of time, lost weight and had better insulin and cholesterol measures, whereas the mice who ate whenever they wanted, known as "ad libitum" eating (which is like human grazing) became obese and diabetic.

These results were shocking, and, importantly, repeatable. They triggered a whole new avenue of intermittent fasting research – intermittent because you switch between eating by day and fasting by night.

The next stop on the research trail was to find out what

the usual eating pattern of Americans was like in the 21st century. How closely are we actually following the three-meal-a-day paradigm many of us were brought up on in the twentieth century? How like the *ad libitum* mice who became obese and diabetic are we in our eating patterns nowadays?

Suddenly, rather than blaming millions of people around the world for being obese and diabetic because of *what* they were eating, maybe part of the problem was the *timing and frequency* of eating? Are those overnight stretches between meals in our eating schedules, which used to be practised in the first three quarters of the twentieth century (before constant access to food via takeaways and 24-hour supermarkets), key to helping us get away with all the ultra-processed junk we consume?

A potential problem is that in modern-day society few of us are making use of the power of fasting and switching on the mechanisms which could heal and help us thrive. This is because many of us are eating and drinking from the moment we wake until late at night, when we switch off the laptop/iPad/phone and slump asleep, as researchers soon found out.

The Salk Institute in San Diego, which undertook the mice studies described above, decided to look in detail at the average eating patterns of humans.

They armed a group of people with 'feedograms' for three weeks. This is where individuals use their smartphones to photograph all eating and drinking events, which are then beamed to a server with timestamp and location managed by researchers. Every crisp/biscuit crumb/dark chocolate square had to be declared. The subjects were also randomly messaged at different points in the day asking if they had eaten in the past 30 minutes and could reply yes or no. This helped sweep up any forgotten reporting on the photo front. The subjects were people who believed that they were eating three times a day over about 12 hours.

However, as you might have guessed, that wasn't what was happening in reality.

The study found that subjects were having between 4.2 and 15.52 eating events a day and spreading food and beverages over almost 15 hours daily – very different to three times over 12 hours, which had been the participants' perception. Every food or drink containing one calorie or more counted as an event. More than half of participants were eating or having a drink of some description hourly. The digestive system was constantly on go-go-go, digesting and dealing with edible substances either in chewable or liquid form (e.g. alcohol) and switching on all the hormones, digestive juices and energy the body needs to digest. The only time their bodies had a rest from eating and digesting was when they briefly slept. Their bodies never received a fully restorative long fast.

The same clinic report also asked a small group of overweight and obese people to eat in a 10-hour time slot each day, which resulted in an average 3.2 kg weight loss (about 7 pounds) over 16 weeks. This was without counting a single calorie or changing the American diet itself. This indicated that eating in a 10-hour slot may be effective and manageable for humans, and therefore was a timing pattern to develop going forward (rather than an eight-hour or nine-hour time slot, which was considered more difficult for people to comply with for long). Further studies also started showing that time-restricted eating improved the function of the pancreas (responsible for insulin control) and lowered blood pressure. The studies on mice had successfully translated to humans.

This is the point at which, if the world was a better place, millions of dollars would have been funnelled quickly into human research leading to lots of big-population studies. If the timing of when you eat could sort out global problems like obesity, type 2 diabetes and heart attacks, we should get big data and share the news with everyone. In England, 63% of adults are overweight or obese, according to National Health Service figures released in 2020, a figure which rose steeply between 1993 and 2000. In the US, latest figures show that 71% of the adult population is obese or overweight. Cheap, simple solutions are vital. Right?

The issue with TRE is that there is no crock of gold at the end of the rainbow. There is no multi-billion-dollar drug to sell. Sharing with people the news that regimenting the timing of meals may reverse some big problems isn't going to make pharmaceutical companies rich. It could actually make pharmaceutical companies poorer, as sales of bariatric equipment, insulin-controlling drugs and blood-pressure medications could go down if we all practised eating in a 10-hour time slot each day.

Human studies in the lead-up to 2021 are finally flourishing beyond small specialist groups of people, and finding that the power of eating for 10 hours a day and fasting for 14 can empower you to boost your health.

Here is a round-up of some of the most recent studies from labs showing us why eating in a 10-hour time slot is effective.

In a clinical report by Wilkinson et al in the journal *Cell Metabolism* in 2020, 19 people suffering from metabolic syndrome ate in a 10-hour time slot each day. Metabolic syndrome, also known as Syndrome X, is the medical term used when a cluster of obesity, type 2 diabetes and heart disease is seen in one person (see box 1.1 for a full explanation and to see if you have metabolic syndrome, or early signs of it). There has been a lot of mention recently in the press of metabolic syndrome, as it raises your vulnerability to Covid-19.

Sixteen of the subjects were walking pharmacies (known in the medical world as 'polypharmacy patients', taking several pharmaceutical drugs for multiple abnormalities). The participants had already tried calorie-controlled diets and exercise programmes to try to reduce their weight, without success.

For three months they were asked to eat and drink in a 10-hour time slot each day. They were only allowed water, or to take their drugs, outside that slot. Unlike some previous TRE studies, these people could choose early TRE or late TRE. This is thought to have helped compliance, as people could choose an option that better suited their physiology (e.g. if they are naturally hungry early in the morning or not) and other commitments.

Early TRE meant eating from 8am and finishing by 6pm.

Late TRE meant opening the eating slot at 10am and finishing by 8pm.

Before the study, most had been spreading their eating and drinking over 14 hours, not 10. They received absolutely no advice about what they should or shouldn't eat, simply to stick to their usual diet. They were instructed only to limit their eating and drinking to the chosen 10-hour slot. Compliance was good; they strayed from timings by more than one hour on average just once a fortnight.

These were the results (and bear in mind they had one 'cheat' day every fortnight):

Weight

They lost on average 3kg (6.6 pounds – which is almost half a stone) and developed a better body composition, seeing a 4% reduction in waist measurement on average, with 3% from the organs around the middle of the body. This type of fat, known as 'visceral fat', is particularly dangerous as it can raise your risk of heart disease and type 2 diabetes, so a method that can reduce this particular area is held in high esteem. (Visceral fat is measured using something called bioelectrical impedance, which sends currents through the body.) The authors noted that losing half a pound a week, which is what happened here, is similar to some calorie-controlled diets over three months, but with those you don't get the heart health improvements, which we'll come to in a minute. Another observation from me: subjects didn't even have to give up their favourite foods.

Heart

Significant reductions in blood pressure (average systolic by 4%, average diastolic by 8%) and their cholesterol scores improved.

Diabetes

Fasting glucose and insulin measurements improved. HbA1c – a standard marker you'll often see on GP blood panels to check for diabetes – improved. See box below for details on how to get your own markers checked.

Interestingly, the more out of range the subjects' markers had been at the start of the study, the better the results. There was also the question of whether the timing of eating had helped reset the subjects' internal clocks (their circadian rhythms – see box on page 9), which in turn may have improved their response to their drugs. Many participants reported they slept much better (longer and more deeply), even though this hadn't been one of the initial measures of the study.

How do we know these results weren't a fluke?

In a small randomised controlled trial in the publication *Obesity* in 2020 (by Chow et al), 20 overweight people were split into two groups. One group carried on eating for at least 15 hours a day, while the other half were asked to only eat during eight hours of the day for three months. Interestingly, most TRE participants managed to fit their eating into 10 hours a day, so the actual results should be viewed as being based on 10-hour eating. A smartphone app was used to check compliance.

Among the TRE group, obese people were told to eat between 9am and 5pm or 12pm and 8pm – but, as mentioned, they ate in 10-hour slots when it came to actual day-in, day-out practice during the study. The latest they could eat was 8pm. The other group just continued eating normally any time they wanted. Both groups had no advice from the researchers about the actual content of their diet.

The TRE group lost weight (an average of 3.6kg, which is almost 8 pounds, or just over half a stone) and visceral fat went down by 11%. They also had improved heart stats (triglycerides, a marker of heart health, for example, went down by an average of 23%) and better blood sugar control (fasting glucose went down by 7.7%), meaning they were less likely to develop type 2 diabetes.

The non-TRE group, the people spreading their eating over 15 hours or more, lost 1.5kg, which is just over 3 pounds, but the amount of visceral fat stayed the same. Both groups had to photograph their food on a smart phone and answer random texts asking if they had eaten in the past half an hour. The non-TRE group's fasting glucose saw insignificant change, and triglycerides remained the same.

So, what happens when we look at timing of eating in larger populations?

A study in 2019 in the publication *Nutrients* (by Ha and Song) analysed 24-hour food diaries of 14,279 Korean people. The researchers looked at associations between the times of day that people ate and whether they suffered from obesity, heart disease or type 2 diabetes.

The researchers found:

- Men and women who front-loaded their eating to earlier in the day (the 'morning eaters') were less overweight, diabetic and heart-diseased.
- Men and women who ate after 9pm (classified as 'night eaters') had more prevalence of weight gain, diabetes and heart measurements out of range than non-night eaters.
- The big surprise in this study was this: individuals who had long overnight fasts (more than 12 hours) but insufficient sleep (less than six hours per night) were associated with a high risk of weight gain, diabetes and heart disease.

This is where the research is beginning to get really interesting and supports some of the cases I've seen in my clinic, where gentler fasting has proved better than long and harsh. Some people drive themselves hard to eat in a smaller window of time, for example eight or six hours a day (meaning a fast of 16 or even 18 hours over the 24-hour day). Some do what is known as 8:16 for months (eat for eight hours, fast for sixteen), the belief being that the longer the fast, the better the results will be. This Korean study shows us that longer and harder isn't always better. If your fasting isn't backed up by making sleep a priority, you could end up sicker and heavier.

Another study, this time in *Cell Metabolism* in 2020 (by

Cienfuegos et al), also indicated that longer fasts don't produce better results. Researchers arranged people into groups: some could eat in a challenging four-hour slot (3–7pm) and others in a six-hour 1–7pm slot, for eight weeks. They were allowed water and zero-calorie coffees and teas during their fasts. Interestingly, the weight loss and improved diabetes markers were very similar in both groups. Although this study wasn't testing a 10-hour window specifically, the experiment does indicate that despite what you might think logically, longer fasting isn't necessarily better.

This is why researchers and clinicians like me are discovering that there is a 'sweet spot' with TRE. Our bodies always want to get into balance – which is called homeostasis. Our physiology is constantly trying to get back to a healthy default position, like a thermostat on the central heating keeping our home comfortable – not sweltering-hot or freezing cold. In my experience in my clinic, I have found there is a delicate line in finding the right length of comfortable and gentle fast for you to switch on the benefits of fasting for your weight, heart and insulin balance, without depleting the body and feeling awful.

Fasting can be our saviour if used carefully – when we have more than 12 hours without food, a 'metabolic switch' gets turned on in the body, helping us thrive and survive. It is thought that the first couple of hours after these 12 hours may be the most useful ones to our body, hence eating in a 10-hour time slot and fasting for 14 hours overnight is a practical way to get benefits without hardship.

I've been honing eating by day and overnight fasting for

several years, trying different combinations with hundreds of clients – at my group workshops in London, health retreats in Ibiza and Menorca, one-to-one clinics in Harley Street and Mayfair, VIP home visits and, more recently, on my Zoom clinics with clients from around the world. I receive referrals from private GPs, gastroenterologists, psychiatrists and rheumatologists, among others, as well as self-referrals from people who have often found me through my book *The Gut Makeover*, published in 2015. I first discovered the initial seeds of the idea of TRE reading mice studies ahead of writing my gut book. I was intrigued by how the mice's microbiomes (gut bacteria connected with the health of many other systems in the body) thrived and became healthier when they had a pause from eating lasting between 12 and 16 hours. I started to tentatively try 12-hour fasting with clients who were open to this, to see if it would improve their digestive health. It often did.

Since then I've worked together with clients using this new 10-hour timing to support a wide range of issues, with weight loss being a welcome result or side effect. As we've seen, the research on TRE was initially based on mice studies, and has more recently been proven to work in humans for weight loss, improved heart health and blood sugar balance. But eating in a 10-hour slot and having an overnight 14-hour fast in my experience can help reset many other systems in the body too. Some of these mechanisms are explained further in Chapter 2.

Studies to specifically test if 10-hour TRE can help with other conditions beyond weight, heart health and preventing diabetes are still scarce, but here I can share with you some of the issues I have seen 10-hour TRE help with, probably through a process called autophagy, where the body goes into repair mode when it has a long stretch without food. For example:

- Irritable Bowel Syndrome (IBS) – constipation, loose stools or a mixture of both
- Acid reflux
- Small Intestinal Bacterial Overgrowth (SIBO)
- Inflammatory Bowel Disease (IBD e.g. Crohn's and Ulcerative Colitis)
- Diverticulitis
- Skin conditions including the herpes virus, acne, eczema and psoriasis
- Better sleep, which in turn helps dial down anxiety

A lot of the work I do is helping to motivate people to make small changes to their daily eating pattern, and brainstorming where to tweak and personalise timings to get results. In this book I will share lots of my experience working with people like you from all walks of life, and all parts of the world, to improve health using this very simple and effective method. I've seen it help people on benefits as well as billionaires. You don't need to be wealthy to access it – you can access my experience and knowledge right here. There is potentially much to gain from these small and safe changes done correctly.

Since the early TRE studies, many people, off their own backs, have logically jumped on the idea of time-restricted eating and started practising it. TRE is safe and cheap, and you don't have anything to lose by trying it. However, what I have learnt in my clinical practice using the 10-Hour Diet with hundreds of real people, in real life, is that to get results, the devil is in the detail of application. The internet is awash with conflicting views on TRE. This is why I have written this book. It means all the most up-to-date science, plus my experience working with this method successfully and honing it to real life, are shared with you here, so you can find a pattern that works for you to reach your health goals.

I'm writing this book so you can find your 10-Hour Diet sweet spot.

Summary: What the science is telling us . . .

- Eating for 10 hours and fasting for 14 hours is likely the sweet spot in humans; eating in a shorter window and fasting for longer may not necessarily bring more benefits.
- The consensus is that 8pm (or earlier for some people) is a healthy cut-off for consuming food (stopping 2–3 hours before bed), when the body is primed to handle food better.
- The more overweight and out of range the health markers, the greater the results of eating in a 10-hour time slot.
- Consuming your biggest meal earlier in the day (or 'frontloading') is best for some people, while eating more later can be most effective for others. Choosing the one that you feel suits you personally can help you comply better.

- You can probably cheat once a fortnight and still get results.
- You can keep eating your normal background diet and get results just by adjusting the timings over three months.
- Photographing or journaling what you're eating and keeping a record of timings can help keep you on track.
- Prioritising time to sleep is essential to get great results, and, in turn, eating in a 10-hour time slot may actually help improve the quality of your sleep.

HOW CAN WE LOSE WEIGHT WITHOUT COUNTING CALORIES?

What are the mechanisms behind the 10-Hour Diet? These are the current theories on why eating in a 10-hour timeslot can lead to weight loss:

1. **A restricted window for eating = fewer calories**
   In mice studies, the mice didn't have fewer calories. Only the timings of access to food changed, and the ones eating in restricted blocks of time lost weight. In human studies, although people were encouraged to eat their usual diet, there was a natural reduction by some in calories overall (about 20%). This is because cutting off eating by, say, 8pm meant people didn't

consume as much alcohol or snacks on the sofa in the evening.

2. **The 10-Hour Diet makes us less hungry**

   The hormones that signal to us that we are full up – the gut hormones PYY (peptide YY), GLP-1 (glucagon-like peptide-1) and GIP (gastric inhibitory polypeptide) – go up.

   A hormone that signals to us that we are hungry – e.g. ghrelin – goes down.

   When we are eating round the clock, e.g. 15 hours a day (instead of 10), these hormones can become dysregulated, making us feel hungry all the time, and rarely full up. Giving your body 14 hours to fast allows your hunger hormones to get back into balance so we don't feel hungry all the time and we receive the message clearly when we are full up.

3. **Food eaten earlier in the day gets burnt off more**

   Moving around all day will naturally offset the front-loaded calories, whereas food eaten close to bedtime has less chance to burn.

4. **TRE promotes fat-burning**

   After about 12 hours without food, the body has used up stored sugar from the liver and starts to burn fat for energy in the morning until we start eating.

Overnight fasting (12 hours or more) also promotes 'metabolic flexibility', inducing special enzymes and hormones, so the fat-burning machinery of the body functions optimally.

5. **TRE reduces the fat-storage hormone insulin**
   When you fast for more than 12 hours, your insulin falls, preventing fat storage.

WHAT *DID* SUBJECTS USUALLY CONSUME DURING THEIR OVERNIGHT FASTS?

- Lots of water
- In some studies, black coffee and tea (no milk, no sugar) were also allowed
- Their prescription drugs

WHAT IS A CIRCADIAN RHYTHM?

We are naturally programmed to work in sync with the Earth's natural cycles of light and darkness.

Light goes through our pupils and tells our body to perform certain functions and release hormones (chemical messengers) and enzymes to digest and absorb food and be active by day.

In darkness, the body produces hormones to help us sleep and for the body to repair.

For this reason, eating after sundown is a big ask for our digestive system, and some hormones just don't function at full throttle at this time. This explains why so many people have digestive issues after they've eaten late at night.

Because some hormones are designed to work optimally earlier in the day, eating earlier will mean you digest and burn food better, which means there is less risk of becoming overweight and diabetic – both of which are more likely with later-evening eating.

Eating at regular times within a 10-hour slot during the daytime sends powerful messages to your body to do all its circadian-rhythm functions in an orderly and healthy manner, as it is designed to do.

Eating erratically at different times of day and night does the opposite – disrupting the normal function of hormones such as insulin and hunger hormones such as ghrelin, making you feel hungry a lot of the time, leading to weight gain and the risk of becoming diabetic.

For this reason, it is better to have your highest-calorie meal earlier in the day, rather than late at night. The 10-Hour Diet can have a positive impact on the functioning of your circadian rhythm and therefore optimal functioning of all the organs in your body.

Here are some interesting areas controlled by the clock in your brain and the peripheral ones in your organs which are influenced by cycles of light and darkness, and by times of eating:

- Your body produces the right amount of insulin during daylight. This is the hormone made by your pancreas to carry food, which is broken down into sugar, around the body either to be used as energy or, if you aren't busy, to be laid down as fat.
- Athletic performance is best in the late afternoon – which is important to know if you are a professional athlete or in a competitive sport.
- Blood pressure is lowest when sleeping and rises on waking, and is highest during the day.

SUGAR, INSULIN CONTROL AND TYPE 2 DIABETES EXPLAINED

How a healthy body handles sugar

When we are healthy, we eat food and it is broken down in our digestive system by stomach acid and enzymes into small particles which pass through the sieve-like barrier of our gut into our bloodstream. A hormone called insulin is produced from a small leaf-shaped organ called the pancreas. Insulin is pumped into our bloodstream to help make energy from sugar if we are busy, or to lay it down as fat if we're not.

If we eat two or three times a day in a 10-hour window, sugar and insulin levels rise after eating and then fall. When we stop eating and when we sleep, sugar and insulin have a chance to fall. This means the pancreas has a rest and can repair itself, and our cells have a break, too, from being flooded with insulin.

How an unhealthy body might handle sugar

If we eat little and often, up to 15 times a day from the moment we wake until we go to bed (common in today's society), sugar levels and insulin levels remain chronically raised. The pancreas is demanded to pump out insulin continually with little break. If we eat late at night, the pancreas is being asked to produce insulin at a time of day when it should be resting. It has clock genes in it which programme it to work at full steam during the daytime. If we chronically eat little and often and well into the night, there are two irregularities that might occur in some people. Either the pancreas stops producing as much insulin, or stops altogether ('I'm going on strike, I'm knackered!!'). This can lead to levels of sugar remaining high in the blood stream, causing damage to blood vessels. This is the reason untreated type 2 diabetes can become so dangerous, and can go on to cause blindness, toes having to be amputated, or heart attacks. Alternatively, our cells can become what is called 'insulin resistant'. This means they stop insulin from penetrating their walls, which in turn causes sugar and insulin to remain dangerously high in the bloodstream, creating damage in the body. Insulin resistance can occur before someone becomes fully diabetic (when the pancreas can't produce so much insulin anymore). A sign that someone is pre-diabetic can be when a blood test shows that their sugar and insulin remain high even after an overnight fast. A blood measure of insulin resistance is Hba1C – see below on how to get this measured and monitored.

DO I HAVE METABOLIC SYNDROME?

Take a look at the following statements:

1. I have belly fat: my waist measures more than 85cm if I'm a woman and more than 90cm if I'm a man (see box below with details of how to measure this accurately).
2. I have high blood pressure (defined as systolic reading above 130mmHg or diastolic above 85mmHg).
3. I have low HDL-cholesterol (under 1.3mmol/L or 40mg/dl for men and under 1.3mmol/L or 50mg/dl for women).

4. I have high triglycerides (above 1.7mmol/L or 150mg/dl).
5. I have high fasting glucose (above 5.6mmol or 100mg/dl).

Note: *You will find these figures vary slightly between the different organisations who put together the definitions – I've picked the entry-level, most moderate figures for diagnosis.*

If three or more of these statements apply to you, you suffer from metabolic syndrome.

Remember, the Wilkinson study showed that eating in a 10-hour time slot pre-8pm daily for three months helped reduce weight and blood pressure, and improved heart markers as well as glucose and insulin measures in people with metabolic syndrome. So, if you have it, the 10-Hour Diet could help.

You can find the numbers above on standard blood panels performed by your GP. The next time you have a blood test, ask for a copy of the actual results. Many surgeries only release them if there is a number out of range, and only if they are out of range on their particular scales, which can vary from country to country, health provider to health provider. However, getting hold of the latest panel, and seeing which direction your figures are going in, even if they aren't out of range yet, can be extremely useful, and motivating for managing your own health and keeping healthy. For one, it will give you a sense of how urgently you need to make 10-hour eating a priority, and it can also help you get your family and friends on side to help protect your health.

Many companies offer annual health checks for employees over 40 years old, and these markers are usually measured in those. So, if you have access to a company programme, use it to track these figures.

HOW TO MEASURE YOUR WAIST ACCURATELY

This is likely to be more accurate if you ask someone to help you . . .

Lift clothing.

Hold the tape measure halfway between your lowest rib and the top of your hip bones, just above your belly button.

Wrap the tape measure around your body, ending up half way between your lowest rib and the top of your hip bone back where you started. Make sure the tape measure is straight on both sides.

Breathe out and take the measurement with the tape measure – not tight, not too slack.

Repeat again to make sure the measurement you had is repeatable and therefore likely to be the right one!

WHO SHOULD AVOID THIS DIET AND WHO SHOULD SEEK ADVICE FROM THEIR DOCTOR?

The 10-Hour Diet is not recommended for anyone with a history of eating disorders.

It is not recommended if you are already a type 1 or type 2 insulin-dependent diabetic unless closely monitored by a medically qualified doctor.

This diet could help prevent type 2 diabetes developing or, according to studies, may reverse early signs. If using this diet in the early signs of out-of-range blood sugar levels, talk to your doctor before trying it.

If you are taking prescription drugs, make sure you are checking in regularly with the doctor or consultant who has prescribed them while you are following this diet. Never change your medication doses or frequency yourself without direct consultation from the doctor who has prescribed them.

CHAPTER TWO

The Power of the 10-Hour Diet

So, what are the potential results from the 10-Hour Diet? What is the power of eating in a 10-Hour time slot and fasting for 14?

When we do this, we switch on multiple mechanisms in the body which will help us lose weight and live longer.

This switch, known as 'the metabolic switch', flicks on after around 12 hours of fasting. This is why having a break from any calories for 14 hours in the 24-hour clock can be really smart. A lot of the magical repair in the body takes place between the 12- and 14-hour mark without food.

For best results, a 10-hour-eating time slot needs to be followed by 14 hours overnight without food, alcohol, or any kind of calorie or artificial sweetener.

Here is a summary of systems in your body which benefit from the magic of eating for 10 hours and fasting for 14, which can be achieved simply by making small and significant changes to the timings of your meals. For many people, it simply means eating breakfast a little later and supper slightly earlier.

Potential results

Body fat

Fasting for 14 hours can aid fat loss without making major dietary changes, and in time help you feel less hungry. It can increase the metabolic rate and help you burn more energy from food eaten in the daytime (called the thermic effect).

Heart

Fasting can reduce blood pressure (if too high), and other cardio markers, such as cholesterol and triglycerides, can also improve.

Brain

Fasting has been proven in mice to increase production of Brain Derived Neurotrophic Factor (BDNF), a substance that helps protect the brain from dementia and makes it more malleable, called 'plasticity'. When the brain is more plastic, it works better, so you are sharper and your mood is better too.

Pancreas

When you're fasting, cells are repaired, so production of the hormone insulin normalises (not too much, not too little). This can mean that cells of the body handle insulin better, so you are protected against type 2 diabetes. This organ will also help you digest food more efficiently when in good order, as it has to produce two and a half litres of enzymes which help break down food each day (see below).

The digestive system

The lining of the digestive tract and the stomach produce enzymes (as does the pancreas, above). The stomach also produces acid to break down food each day. Every time we see or smell food, the digestive system starts gushing with these enzyme and acid juices – totalling between five and nine litres per person per day. When we give it a break from lots of traffic (food) at night, the lining of the digestive tract has a chance to repair itself. Eating by day and fasting by night can thereby help improve symptoms of digestive disorders.

Gut microbiome

The trillions of bacteria in the digestive system that make up what we call the microbiome (now classified as a whole organ in itself) can thrive and diversify when you give them a break from eating and drinking relentlessly. A healthy microbiome can improve Irritable Bowel Syndrome (IBS) symptoms such as bloating, irregular stools and gas and also communicates with your brain, immune system and heart to be healthy.

Immune system

Fasting results in a reduction of inflammatory cytokines, meaning less inflammation in the body (think of any chronic inflammatory condition in the body, from asthma or arthritis, to eczema and dermatitis). Fasting can make your immune system act in a healthy manner and stave off illness without becoming disordered and attacking the cells of your own body (called auto-immunity).

Liver

In a break from eating, the liver rebuilds its cells so we can detoxify all the nasties that come into our bodies, from fumes in the air to pesticides in our foods. Our liver is a mini laundrette. When the toxins going into our body are made safe and efficiently eliminated through stools, benefits range from clearer skin to less risk of cancer.

Sleep

Some research has shown improved sleep as one of the unexpected added bonuses of eating by 8pm within a 10-hour eating slot. One reason for that could be because people have less opportunity to drink alcohol in the evening, the consumption of which leads to shallower, less restorative sleep.

Exercise

When we finish eating, say in the early evening, the body breaks down the calories consumed and uses them to power our sleep, digestion, brain power (our dreams!) and repair us.

The body needs a lot of energy just to go about powering basic living, breathing and sleeping. After this meal has been fully digested, broken down and made into sugar to fuel us during the first few hours of sleep, the body then has to find some more sugar to keep going.

This is when it will signal to the liver to release stored sugar called glycogen. I like to think of this like a safe being cracked open and the loot being released to be enjoyed. After all the glycogen has been spent, the body then has to look elsewhere for fuel.

At this point, usually around 12 hours into a fast, your body turns to its fat stores, which start to be broken down and burnt as energy, powering your basic living and breathing. If you happen to be moving when it does this, your body will burn even more fat. This is why every minute between the 12th and 14th hour before starting your 10 hours of eating is really important.

If you are healthy, and you want to boost fat-burning during those two special hours, you could do exercise. Exercising on an empty stomach first thing in the morning may sound unorthodox, but it can be effective for some people's weight loss. Research shows that exercise in the fasted state can enhance muscle growth and endurance (however, if you have any health conditions please do check with your GP first).

Some people might feel a little unenergized exercising this way if they are used to having a banana or some quick sugars beforehand, as you'll be exercising on ketones – chemicals made in the liver when you are burning fat.

You don't have to force yourself down to a gym and start

pumping iron to get benefits. Any kind of movement during your 14-hour fast will help burn fat. So, if you normally eat breakfast at home, what about eating a bit later at work? This may buy you another hour of fasting and you get the added benefit of boosting your fat-burning while getting to the car/on the train/walking up the stairs to the office. If you work at home, how about walking round the block before you sit down at your computer to spend some extra fat? You could do some very simple exercises at home – a few star jumps, stretches, or press-ups. Try a 10-minute yoga or high intensity interval training (HIIT) short free session from the internet. Skip for five minutes if you have a skipping rope. It really can be quick and simple measures that optimise fat spending at this time of day.

WHAT IS AUTOPHAGY?

When we have a 12–14-hour overnight fast, the body goes into a state of autophagy. This is a type of bodily house-keeping where cells are repaired and old cells are slung out. Our organs, such as our heart, brain, liver, gut and skin, are repaired and rejuvenated. In my opinion, there really isn't any potion, lotion or pill you can buy that's as powerful as a proper overnight fast for keeping us youthful and protecting us against heart attack, dementia, digestive issues, cancer and looking our best.

EARLY TRE OR LATE TRE – WHICH IS BETTER?

Eating earlier in the day may be more effective to protect us from type 2 diabetes and heart disease than eating later in the day.

This was the finding of a 2018 *Cell Metabolism* study, by Sutton et al, looking at pre-diabetic people eating three meals between 9am and 3pm and comparing results with those eating three meals in a 12-hour stretch (e.g. 8am to 8pm) each day.

Subjects eating all their meals before 3pm improved their insulin sensitivity. This is thought to be because eating was aligned with our circadian rhythm – when insulin is influenced by the natural cycles of light in the day to handle food best.

The take-away from this study: if you are pre-diabetic, eat your main meal of the day at breakfast or lunch, when insulin can handle food better.

The same study also saw blood pressure improve in the early-eating group, meaning that if you have high blood pressure, eating your main meal earlier in the day may help normalise your blood pressure more than if you eat your main meal later in the day, which could disrupt it.

CHAPTER THREE

Changing Behaviour

When I was a child in Britain in the seventies, mealtimes were anchors. I often talk to my clients about the differences between then and now in terms of how we eat, as I believe the changes in society have contributed to the rising obesity figures.

Think about it. I don't know about everyone else, but in my family, every day was the same. Breakfast: 8am at home. Lunch: 12.30 at school. Supper: 6pm at home. By 6.30 we had finished eating; we cleared the table and my parents washed up. My mum would close the kitchen door and our evening would begin. I remember the frosted vertical glass of the kitchen clouding the sight of the kitchen interior, strip lights out. The eating day had ended. We then had a natural fast from 6.30pm to 8am the next day – 13 and a half hours where the body had a chance to reset itself.

It was a traditional 1970s gig. We ate together as a family, and you were banned from eating between meals so that you 'wouldn't ruin your appetite'. Around 5pm I would get very hungry (often I hadn't eaten enough school lunch because they had served something I didn't like) and, despite pestering my mum, would have to wait until 6pm to eat. Of course, there were exceptions, but our routine was pretty much the same every day. Snacking was frowned upon and, in any case, opportunities for it were scant.

A regimented pattern of timings for eating and a lack of snacking was pretty usual in the UK in the late sixties and early-to-mid-seventies. Food had to be planned, prepared and cooked at home most of the time – not to mention physically purchased in a shop between 9am and 5pm Monday to Friday, and 9am and 2pm on Saturdays. Many shops also closed on Thursday afternoons to make up for them having to work Saturday mornings.

Compare this to today's world: of 24-hour supermarkets; where you can have any snack you want, delivered at the touch of a button, 24/7; where junk food is subtly marketed at us wherever we go – product placement in TV shows, or strategically placed by the till in a petrol station. We're manipulated to snack without even realising we're doing it.

And now, obesity and diabetes rates are sky high: 63% of us are overweight or obese in the UK; 71% in the US.

BLOOD SUGAR MANTRA

Many nutritionists (including me) and medics have been taught in their training about the importance of blood-glucose balance. We were told that humans should eat little and often to prop up the levels of sugar in the blood stream to help avoid type 2 diabetes and obesity. This learning has been turned on its head by TRE research.

We are now discovering that eating multiple times around the clock without much break could be part of the problem, rather than the solution. Eating little and often means you have to produce a lot of insulin all day long. Insulin is a fat-storage hormone, and a pancreas that is producing insulin on and off all day long can become a very tired pancreas, leading to type 2 diabetes.

A recent study of almost 49,000 postmenopausal women found that those eating four times a day, instead of one to three times, were associated with a 36% higher risk of type 2 diabetes. The authors hypothesised that the idea of keeping blood glucose and insulin steady (to avoid highs and lows) may actually be placing extra stress on the pancreas and raising the risk of diabetes rather than lowering it. Imagine how much insulin the subjects in the Salk Institute studies were producing who were eating 15 times a day!

The blood sugar balance theory has led many of us to develop a fear of being stranded without food, suffering a blood sugar dip leading to low energy, shaking, brain fog and bad mood.

These symptoms really do exist in anyone whose insulin is uncontrolled – ask anyone who suffers blood sugar dips. I was one of them. Sometimes it would even happen after eating a big meal, as my handling of insulin and sugar was clearly messed up.

I used to eat little and often, and my handbag always contained nuts and seeds to keep my blood sugar topped up without sudden plunges. It was pretty inconvenient. I'd be sitting in lecture halls trying to dull the sound of the crackling nut packet and to chew without being rude.

I often meet clients who show me food diaries which contain six feedings a day. Breakfast within half an hour of getting up. Morning snack. Lunch. Afternoon snack. Dinner. Bedtime snack. Many, like the old me, live in complete fear of a blood sugar crash, so eat from waking to sleeping – spreading out their eating over 16 hours rather than 10. My mum would be turning in her grave.

When I first started reading the scientific literature around TRE and fasting for 14 hours a night (instead of my usual eight), I was frightened and found it very difficult to accept. With nutrition, however, you have to have an open mind to new research – it's part of the job.

I was convinced I would wake up shaking with hunger in the morning – getting up and almost fainting and seeing stars if I stopped the bedtime oatcake snacks.

Little did I know that eating so many times a day was confusing my hormones and putting strain on my pancreas. I was eating over so many hours that my hunger hormones (such as ghrelin, which tells you when you're hungry), was probably all over the place.

So when I started to experiment with overnight fasting and eating in a 10-hour window, I found that before bed I was a bit peckish in the first week. Strangely, despite going to bed hungry the first few days, I was waking up *not* hungry. This was really odd, because before doing long overnight fasts I used to wake up starving.

After about a week of dropping the bedtime snack, the bedtime hunger disappeared as my hunger hormones reset. I started waking up not hungry either, and was having to wait for my hunger hormones to kick in and tell me to eat.

Now that I often eat in a 10-hour window and fast for 14 overnight, I often have no need to carry snacks around with me and I no longer suffer blood sugar crashes.

Revolutionary.

No, *evolutionary.*

We evolved from hunter-gatherers. There were long gaps between meals because you had to hunt or forage for your food. There was legwork involved!

We are very simple animals. See food, catch and eat. See food, gather and eat. Our digestive system cranks into action like a machine at the suggestion of food. We produce up to nine litres of stomach acid and enzymes each day to break food down. Most of this starts flooding the digestive system at the mere sight or suggestion of food. Even sounds associated with food can prime us to eat. Remember Pavlov's dogs? That's you and me.

Lockdown lifestyle

The effects of the 2020 Covid-19 lockdown on our health are yet to be fully explored. But one great thing about the 10-Hour Diet is that it's free and easy – and can adapt to almost any change in routine. If you feel that the lockdown has changed the way you move or eat, introducing this 10-hour window can help you retain some structure.

The downside of artificial lighting

Another factor which has changed the natural timing of our eating is access to artificial light after sundown. After all, it's only recently that we've been able to prepare food after dark. For thousands of years we ate during daylight hours, and the overnight fast started automatically when the sun went down.

Eating the main meal of the day in the evening is a very recent, new habit, becoming fashionable among British aristocrats in the 19th century. They could afford lighting in their households to cook and eat, hence the evening-eating fashion began.

As we've seen, the digestive system is primed to naturally operate best during daylight hours. So of course it makes sense that restricting our eating window helps us lose weight: it reduces the effects of the guerrilla marketing and takes us back to straightforward mealtimes – to the way our bodies used to work.

CHAPTER FOUR

Getting Started

I'm a champion of preparation.

If we were going to run the London marathon, would we wake up one morning, put on our trainers and seamlessly run all 26 miles? Without prior training and assessing the route and terrain, we would suffer physical and mental pain and never reach the finishing line. Discouraged, we might not try again. 'Running's not for me!' we'd wail. But, with a little planning and prior warm-up and practice, running might have changed our lives.

Likewise, changing an eating routine takes a bit of preparation. First, we need to have a picture of the landscape we will be working in. We want to set ourselves up for success and to practise before we dive into the new eating pattern ahead.

When I work with a new client on a dietary intervention, I normally take a measure of their default starting position. We need to do that now, so we know exactly where the potentially tricky areas are, where we really are with our timings and exactly which bits need tweaking.

The 10-Hour Diet hinges on making, in many cases, just

small and consistent timing adjustments for maximum results. Assessing exactly where these are going to be in each particular personal case involves measuring the default starting pattern.

Step One

Therefore, as a first step, I recommend keeping a diary of timings for one or two weeks before committing to the 10-Hour Diet for three months (see Chapter 10).

Three months is a long time, I know. But the science shows that by adjusting your routine for 12 weeks, you can see the best results. So, before we rush into it, I usually ask my clients to record everything they eat and drink for at least one week, so we can be on the lookout for patterns.

Some people write their timings on a piece of old-fashioned paper with a pen and stick it on the fridge with a magnet. Others like to use the notes app on their smartphone to get a sense of their usual timings. However you choose to record your week, the aim is to assess how you could reduce your eating window to 10 hours, finishing by 8pm at the latest.

Being accurate on a daily basis about keeping consumption within the 10-hour window is the key to making this diet work for you. So it's very important to be honest about the hours you consumed, and how you could make sure they're all sub-10. However, in the first instance, don't change your behaviour: be as honest as you can, to show you how many hours you are generally eating for now.

The following template may be useful as a starting point – just remember that the start time is when you have the first calorie of food or drink, and the end time recorded is the last mouthful of a calorie (when you finish eating dinner or drinking any drink containing calories).

DATE	START + END TIMES	EATING-SLOT TOTAL	POTENTIAL EDITS + OBSERVATIONS
Monday			
Tuesday			
Wednesday			
Thursday			
Friday			
Saturday			
Sunday			

Once the week is over, look at your notes and have a think about what you observe. For example, did you need both the latte on the way to work at 8am and the glass of wine on the sofa at 9pm? Which one could you cut out, to fit into the 10-hour window? Could you swap any of these drinks to sparkling water or tea without milk? Say two of your social events this week were drinks/dinners out. Could either of these have been moved to lunch on the weekend? Or, on days when you knew you'd be eating late, could you make adjustments to the time you started consuming calories that morning?

Now you can see where the tricky areas may be, decide how to tackle them.

Step Two

Brainstorm what steps you could take for a successful 10-Hour Diet. Here's my list as an example, followed by a template for you to fill in.

- Having a tasty green tea or white tea (my favourite) in my kitchen cupboard, so when I get up I have a nice warm drink which gives me a boost while I shower, walk the dog, tidy up, cycle to work, prolonging my fast until my eating-window opens.
- Letting those I live with know what my eating pattern is and getting their support. Brainstorming eating times to suit us, and accepting and planning when we'll eat together and when we won't.
- Making my overnight fasts easier by not having treats and snacks like dark chocolate and crisps in my cupboards habitually. When they are there, they call me like the bells and Pavlov's dogs. Removing them from the picture means they can't call out to me after my 10-hour eating slot has ended. Instead, they visit our home at weekends to be shared in good company during mealtimes. (I still eat desserts and treats – just within a 10-hour window!)
- Filling up properly at mealtimes. At weekends, if

the main meal is lunch, making it an event to be enjoyed. On weekday evenings, making sure I'm full up before closing the eating slot for the day.

- If I'm working late, taking a break at 6pm to eat my last meal.
- Socialising with friends and family at the weekend during the daytime – in summer, suggesting picnics and barbecues; in winter, having lunches as a group at home.
- Planning to get to bed at a reasonable time, pottering around, avoiding screens and stimulation (e.g. social media) before bed, so getting to sleep is easier. Making sure the room is fully darkened for sleep time. (Studies show that TRE works best in conjunction with quality sleep.)

Now it's your turn . . .

What actions could you take that would help to make the 10-Hour Diet a success for you? List them here:

MY TOP 10 SUPPORTS

1.

2.

3.

4.

5.

6.

7.

8.

9.

10.

Another area to recognise is boredom- or stress-eating. Sometimes we eat late in the evenings because we feel like eating something to pass the time and/or soothe us. Try to recognise when this is happening, and suggest to yourself other actions or kind gifts to yourself that could give you pleasure and help you feel relaxed that don't involve food.

Here are some of the non-food soothers I use after dinner to relax and have a nice experience . . .

- Take a bath of bubble bath with aromatherapy oils or Epsom bath salts, for achy joints, and magnesium (which incidentally can also help with sleep).

- Read a weekend newspaper dribbled through the whole week in the evenings. I can drag the supplements out for days!
- Have a slow walk around the neighbourhood.
- Catch up with friends by phone, sitting somewhere cosy or walking with headphones.
- Bond with family and share and listen to news about each other's days.
- Do an online yoga or meditation practice – there are so many to choose from now; just 10–15 minutes can feel lovely. I especially like doing Yoga Nidra – the floor one – with a nice blanket and a candle.
- Flick through an illustrated cookery book in bed.

Now it's your turn . . .

MY TOP 6 NON-FOOD SOOTHERS

1.

2.

3.

4.

5.

6.

So, you've assessed how long your current eating slot is, brainstormed ideas for editing it down, thought about what supports you can put in place, and decided what non-food treats you could use if needed. Now it's time to get into the nitty-gritty of the 10-Hour Diet, using the full instructions in the next chapter.

CHAPTER FIVE

How to Practise the 10-Hour Diet

The golden rule for this diet is: *you are the boss.*

This is a totally personalised three-month plan, of which you are the architect. I will show you the principles and how to implement them into your busy life for the best results. If you think about diets and humans logically, it is ludicrous that we would ever expect that one diet would fit all. This is why only *you* can work out the best timings for your body with this plan. After all, only you know the intricacies of your daily schedules, and you know your body best. You have to be honest with yourself from the outset to make this lifestyle liveable and therefore make lasting changes.

Another lesson I have learnt, by working with many different individuals, is that no one likes, or finds it helpful, or keeps new habits going for the long term, by being *told* what to do. That's the parent–child model, or spoon-feeding approach. A coaching, adult-to-adult approach, which is what this diet is based on, is more of a guiding whisper in the ear as you find the right direction and gain speed yourself. What I find works best is presenting the science and the principles, explaining the potential benefits, and working with you to think about your day and your resources, in order to design a way of eating that will suit you and your lifestyle best. For example, there's no point in me telling you to eat your dinner at 6pm if you are on a packed train at that time, but you could think of how you could change your eating pattern somehow to get the benefits of this plan. For example, you could weigh up the cost (in terms of the initial slight discomfort in doing something different to your norm) of pushing your main meal to earlier in the day, and evaluate if the potential benefits make it worth doing.

I have outlined earlier in this book all the benefits of the 10-Hour Diet. I hope to have convinced you that making a few simple changes over the next few weeks and laying down new habits is worth focusing on and practising, because it will improve your quality of life for the long term. So, here goes . . .

The core principles of this three-month diet are:

Eat within a 10-hour time slot during the day.

Fast for 14 hours overnight.

Try to have your last mouthful of food by 8pm at the latest (though some people find 6pm or 7pm to be even more effective).

How it works: two case studies

Of course, eating better-quality food can only boost your health, but this book is not about *what* you eat; it's about *when*.

TRE studies are based on people eating their normal diet and just changing their timings for health benefits.

That said, there's no reason you can't use the focus on timings to also make a few small upgrades to quality of diet, too, if you can. This is merely the icing on the cake, however – you can just focus on timings if that is all you have the capacity for.

Another bonus of this diet is that eating earlier means that, for many people, after a week or so of practise your appetite is reduced in the evening, which means you drink less alcohol and eat fewer snacks.

Here is an example of how someone might eat before starting the 10-Hour Diet:

Case 1

8am: *Cappuccino at home*
10am: *Oat bar at work*
1pm: *Fish and chips in the canteen, followed by a vending machine bar of chocolate*
4pm: *Bag of crisps and a small piece of birthday cake from a colleague*
8.30pm: *Dinner of salmon, asparagus and new potatoes, followed by two pieces of dark chocolate*
9pm: *Finishes eating*

This person is eating in a **13-hour slot: 8am–9pm**.

By changing the cappuccino to a ginger herbal tea, however, we can open the eating window mid-morning – at 10am, at work – instead.

Instead of the sugary oat bar, they might want to introduce a flax and berry shake, which is more filling (see recipe section), taken in a flask to work. By swapping the chocolate bar for an apple, they will also benefit from the fibre and feel even fuller.

Then, after eating an evening meal of similar quality to the one above, they just need to bring dinner forward a little to close the eating slot at 8pm instead of 9pm.

The new eating window is **10am–8pm, following the 10-Hour Diet**, and we've also introduced some good-quality filling foods such as the flaxseeds and fruit.

Starting breakfast two hours later, simply by switching to a hot drink that didn't contain milk, and bringing the end of dinner forward by one hour are all this person needed to do to contain their eating within a 10-hour window.

Let's now look at another example of how someone might eat before the 10-Hour Diet:

Case 2

6.30am: *Shreddies and milk*
1pm: *Sushi with avocado and salmon, followed by a chocolate bar*
10pm: *Fresh pasta and pesto, some chocolate and three glasses of wine*

In this case, eating is spread over a long time – **15.5 hours**, which is almost the whole waking day.

This individual might decide to stop eating breakfast at

home and now has a small bottle of kefir with a banana and a handful of mixed nuts at work when they arrive, at about 8am.

Lunch is at 1pm as before, and they eat a light supper at work at around 5.30pm – usually a varied salad with a piece of satiating protein, which keeps them feeling full all evening.

The new eating window is **8am–6pm, following the 10-Hour Diet**.

At weekends, they might decide to eat a big brunch mid-morning and a roast dinner with lots of vegetables and some roast potatoes with the family mid-afternoon, and a cup of miso later if they are still hungry within their eating window – e.g. at weekends, shifting the eating window two hours forward to **10am–8pm, following the 10-Hour Diet**.

The 10-Hour Diet guidelines

1. Eat two or three proper meals a day in your 10-Hour Diet – and avoid grazing.

Try to have proper meals rather than food and calorie-laden drinks on and off all day, which, according to research, appears to make us heavier and sicker (unless you need to do so regularly for medical reasons).

If you are naturally not a breakfast eater, you may prefer two meals a day with a planned legitimate snack in the middle, if you flag for energy, such as a piece of fresh fruit rather than a handful of nuts. Put them on a plate, sit down and legitimise the snack by chewing properly and mindfully, being present in the moment so you recognise when you are full.

You may find two meals a day with no snacks suits you fine.

If you are a natural breakfast eater, then three meals a day may suit you better; you can choose.

What is key to this diet is self-experimentation. Try what works for you, makes you feel full, and is the right fit for the individual you are. It will make sticking to this approach much easier if you design your own eating pattern.

If you tend to graze when you are stressed, notice when this is happening. Ask yourself how you are feeling when you start reaching or thinking about snacks. As babies, we had a dummy or sucked our thumb to calm down. As adults we often reach for a snack for a calming sensation in the mouth. The mouth is full of sensations. You may find that a glass of water or a warm camomile tea soothes and calms you instead. Or try closing your eyes and breathing deeply for three minutes.

People who fast all the way to lunchtime (the non-breakfast-eaters, who aren't hungry when they wake up) sometimes become aware of bad breath, usually described as smelling like nail varnish remover. This means your body is producing ketone bodies and is therefore definitely burning fat. You can fix this by chewing on cardamom pods and spitting them out (just don't swallow them!).

2. Stop eating between 6pm and 8pm.

Once you have your mealtime pattern worked out (e.g. two meals or three), look at your 10-hour eating slot and decide when you are going to open and close it.

Some people lose more weight finishing by 6pm, some by 8pm. Try out what works better for you. What we know from research is that the later we eat, the more metabolically dangerous for our health it is likely to be. So nudging supper earlier may pay off health-wise.

The eating slot closes when you have eaten and swallowed the last mouthful of food from your day's last meal or liquid containing a calorie. Sometimes people tell me they are 'definitely' eating in a 10-hour time slot of 10am–8pm, but when we go into detail find they aren't. This is because they are *starting* dinner at 8pm and actually finishing at 9pm. It is crucial to success to count the timings from when you finish eating your last meal (or snack!) rather than start.

Your fast isn't a fast if you consume *anything* with calories, no matter how small, during that time. A sip of your partner's wine, or spoonful of ice cream or some popcorn watching telly on the sofa still count! The best results come from closing the eating day between 6pm–8pm and starting the fast at least 2–3 hours before sleep. Consider asking people you live with not to cook delicious food and snacks – or dangle temptation under your nose on the sofa! – after you have closed your eating slot for the day.

3. Stay hydrated during your fast and be careful not to accidentally break it.

The 10-Hour Diet starts when you have the first calorie of the day. So if you put milk in your tea, the 10-Hour Diet has started. Switch to black tea (no sugar), however, and you are still on your overnight 14-hour fast.

Drinks that are OK: Black tea, green tea, white tea, black coffee (if it doesn't have too much of a laxative or jittery effect on you), some herbal teas, water, fizzy water, fizzy water mixed with cooled herbal teas or infused with fresh herbs such as mint). These drinks are all zero calorie so they won't accidentally break your fast. However ... zero-calorie drinks containing artificial sweeteners are not recommended as there are concerns they may make you feel hungrier.

Drinks that aren't OK: any type of tea or coffee with added sugars, milks or artificial sweeteners. Fizzy drinks containing artificial sweeteners or sugar in all its guises.

4. Start your day with movement and/or exercise to burn fat before you eat.

If weight loss is your major goal from this diet, you will have a lot to gain by exercising or simply moving around during the fasted state in the morning before you open your eating slot for the day. This habit does not apply to endurance athletes, who should not exercise in the fasted state as doing so could reduce performance, but is a helpful strategy for us regular people looking to lose a few pounds – although everyone is different, and if you're worried that won't work for you then do check with your GP.

This idea may go against convention, which is to have some quick-releasing sugars such as from a banana before exercise, or a protein bar straight after to provide protein (the building blocks of foods) to help build muscle.

When you wake up in the morning, you need to keep going until you hit the 14-hour-fasted mark. So let's say you finished dinner at 8pm the night before; you are going to want to stay in the fasted state until 10am to enjoy some fat-burning. Or if you finished dinner at 6.30pm and you plan to open your eating window at 8.30am, it is likely that exercising before you eat at 8.30am is going to be the most advantageous time for you to exercise (or walk up the stairs instead of taking the lift) in terms of burning fat for weight loss.

Remember the food from your dinner, and stored sugar in your liver, are likely all burnt up, and the body now switches to burning your stored fat to power you along in the morning. You could just go about your day, commute or chores until you break your fast with breakfast, or you could add in some exercise to burn extra fat.

Studies show us that exercising during the fasted state revs up fat-burning to help weight loss. So although it may seem an uncomfortable idea, at first, to do formal exercise (e.g. an online HIIT class, cycle or run) or walk the stairs to your desk on an empty stomach, there is lots to gain weight-loss-wise from this small tweak to your regime (e.g. not having a banana beforehand or protein bar directly after). Our hunter-gatherer ancestors may have had to spend the first couple of hours each morning on the run for food. We can safely adapt and many people notice their body shape improves doing this. Try it. Although it's not the same for everyone, people often say it is a bit uncomfortable the first few days, and then they don't really notice they haven't eaten once they become accustomed to this practice, and they still build muscle.

If you are someone who is focused on improving your body composition (getting more lean), you may be worried about losing muscle, or not building it, if you don't have that protein bar. As long as you have protein in your 10-Hour Diet somewhere in the day, however, you can build muscle. It doesn't have to be directly before or after you exercise to build it.

A meta-analysis in 2020 – the type of research which pools data from lots of studies and is considered the highest level of evidence – showed it doesn't matter what time of day you eat protein for it to help you build muscle. What is important is that 1) you include protein-rich foods in your diet to build muscle 2) you distribute your protein through your meals throughout the day. The study concluded that immediate pre- or post-protein intake makes no difference to building muscle and strength. In everyday practice this means there is no necessity to rush out of a gym or weight-lifting session and have a protein shake (if that's what you like), a chicken breast or three boiled eggs. If these foods fit your goals for building lean muscle, just have them at your leisure in your meals throughout the day, or later on, when you are ready to open your eating window.

My last tip if you are planning to exercise before opening your 10-hour eating window each day is to stay well-hydrated. Listen to your thirst, have a glass of water or herbal tea soon after waking up, and have more water or herbal teas after exercise. When you do open your eating window a bit later in the morning, after exercise, you could include a banana then or coconut water, or simply put some sea salt on your eggs: bananas, coconut water and sea salt contain electrolytes – the tiny minerals we lose when we sweat and need to replenish during our day for the nervous system to operate well. You could also include berries or cacao for the polyphenols (powerful plant chemicals) in their deep dark colours that fight cancer. See Chapter 6 for two post-workout shakes I have designed for when you are ready to open your eating window if you've exercised in the morning.

5. Include lots of different vegetables and embrace fresh fruit.

You may have heard of the glycemic index at some stage. This is a list of foods with numbers on a scale indicating which ones have a more dramatic impact on blood sugar levels than others. The idea is that foods with a lot of sugar in them or which turn into sugar quickly in the body have higher numbers, and are deemed to be the ones most likely to raise sugar levels in the blood quickly, followed by an insulin response (and potential fat storage), then an energy dip.

We are learning that the glycemic index is a bit pointless for some people because it is based on average responses rather than individual ones. We now know that a food that drives one person's blood sugar high can have little or no impact on another.

In recent years I've noticed people arriving at my clinic fearful of certain fruits, as they have heard about their high GI response. For example, bananas (which contain a wonderful fibre called inulin), mangoes (full of plant chemical flavonoids) and pineapples (containing anti-inflammatory bromelain) are often viewed with horror, based on the GI index numbers. It's a shame, because there are so many hundreds of plant chemicals and fibre in them to feed good bacteria in the gut and make us healthy. Sometimes I feel frustrated when people reject bananas because they have read somewhere that they are high on the GI index, yet their food diary is peppered with chocolate bars – full of harmful, inflammatory types of fat and a range of highly processed sugars that are likely causing much more havoc with health than the odd banana or slice of pineapple. It makes no sense.

Soon we will be able to use gut, blood fat and blood sugar response testing to see which foods are best for the individuals we are. When this happens, you may find that bananas have little impact on your blood sugar levels while someone else has a high response and isn't suited to them. Until we have the technology – ZOE, co-founded by Professor Tim Spector of King's College London and colleagues in the US – observe how you feel after eating higher-sugar fruits such as bananas, mangoes and pineapples. And eat a wide variety of vegetables and fruit to promote a healthy microbiome, which will help you handle sugar better. You may also find that after a week or so practising the 10-Hour Diet that you are better able to tolerate high-sugar fruits as your microbiome gets into a more healthy pattern, which can help you handle sugar better. Intermittent fasting can improve your microbiome, according to latest research. Have fruits cut up into chunks and eaten with all the fibre – the most filling part, which provides food for your gut bacteria to thrive on – rather than juices, where the fibre goes into the bin and just the colourful, sugary water has been extracted. It is likely that we are designed to eat fruits in all their glory, including the fibre, plant chemicals and the natural sugars working in concert together for health.

Another point about fruit and vegetables, now commonly referred to as plants, is that you don't have to turn vegan or fully vegetarian to enjoy the benefits of them. Loading them into whatever existing diet you have can help health, while taking a flexitarian approach can suit others.

6. Plan to succeed by planning what you will eat.

My mum used to ask us what we would like to eat tomorrow, often at the end of a really great family meal together. It used to drive us kids mad. How on earth can you picture what you want to eat tomorrow, or this coming week, when you are brimful of food and the last thing you can imagine is ever eating again?

Now I'm the mum and have the habit of ending a good meal by asking, 'What would you all like to eat tomorrow?' I know that, as the provider of food in the house, one meal ending leaves a gap that needs to be filled with other good ideas ASAP. Otherwise there are wails of teens coming home, opening the fridge and raging: 'Mum, there is absolutely no food in this house!!!'

Often I find the wails of 'there is no food' a bit unfair. I look in the same fridge and see potential meals popping out at me that others haven't pieced together. I look and I see spinach in the freezer, cheese in the fridge, flour and eggs in the cupboards. 'How about spinach pancakes?' I say. Or I bang a few cupboards open and shut and find there are potatoes (which could be slung in the oven for an hour to make jacket potatoes), and could be served with those tasty tinned black beans in chilli sauce, with grated cheese from the fridge door and some sliced avocado that's lying around. Or there's some frozen salmon in the freezer, which could be sautéed in butter with a few sliced almonds and a squeeze of lemon and served with frozen sweet potato chips (which take 20 minutes in the oven).

I now make a list of potential meals for the week and put it up on the wall in the kitchen, spelling out what meals are in the cupboards to make it easier. (I don't put which will be eaten on which days, so we can decide nearer the time what we actually feel like.) Sometimes there are more meals in there than I thought, or I visualise others and realise that with a few additional purchases we are almost there.

Have a think about what you're going to eat each day, and what storecupboard essentials to get in. (See my shortcuts box in Chapter 8 for ideas.) Some people like to plan ahead a day in advance and buy little and often, others a couple of times a week or once a week. Planning means and having tins and frozen foods to hand can help get meals on the table efficiently, meaning you can eat earlier rather than late at night.

One of the most frequent reasons people in my clinic give for why they are regularly eating late at night is that they haven't visualised and planned what to eat, and have to start popping into shops and starting to cook from scratch at the last minute.

To make the 10-Hour Diet as enjoyable as possible, try to make meals a satisfying event to look forward to, rather than mindless fuel-filling all day long. Lay the table. Collect nice crockery and glasses. You don't have to spend a lot – you can sometimes find amazing pieces in charity shops. Fold a nice napkin. Light a candle. Show yourself loving kindness. When you slow down, you may even notice food tastes better.

7. Journal the time you open your 10-Hour Diet each day and when you close it. Seeing the figures can make a big difference to compliance and success.

- Jot down your start and finish times anywhere that suits you – your phone, a notebook, a scrap of paper. You can use the templates in Chapter 10. Seeing the figures can really help you see how adherent to the 10-hour slot you are, spot particular diary events that are sabotaging you, try to tweak your eating on those particular days accordingly, and stay on track. Often people think they are eating in a 10-hour slot, only going off-piste maybe once a fortnight, but when they show me their notes on their phone, we see it's actually off sync more like three times a week, and that explains why the weight or health markers aren't improving much.

- Don't beat yourself up if times are astray as you start practising new timings. Information is power – use what you learn about your eating times to tweak accordingly. (See tools in the journal chapter for more help on this.) In studies, there were times when people went a little off-piste with timings. On average, the timings were out by more than one hour once a fortnight, but people still got great weight loss and metabolic results. So don't beat yourself up if there is a family or work late-night-dining occasion once a fortnight that spoils your diet. Just get back on track as soon as you can.

8. Enlist the support of your friends and family with your new eating times – they may benefit too!

Tell friends and family about your new eating times and get their support.

Other may like to join you too.

Start a WhatsApp group with your household or friends who fancy the 10-Hour Diet too. Take pictures of foods you have found for short cuts and cutting meal-preparation time, or meals which are exciting you.

9. Prioritise sleep.

Key to successfully losing weight with the 10-Hour diet is good sleep. Without good sleep, intermittent fasting can become a strain on the body and be a burden. Good food and good sleep are what restore us and help flick on the metabolic switch to gain overall health benefits from fasting. Make sure you have the obvious basics for sleep covered: try to get digital devices out of your bedroom if they are there and replace with analogue. For stress and busy minds, try one of the many mindfulness apps on the market. Try not to work close to bedtime – potter around and wind down if you can. One of the issues of so much working at home these days is that many of us end up feeling like we live at work. Try to create physical boundaries in your home between work and relaxation.

10. Try to have 20g of protein in your evening meal to curb hunger pangs later in the evening in the first week.

The first week you follow this diet in full, you might feel a little hungry before bed. If you have stopped eating between 6pm and 8pm, it may be several hours before you go to bed.

As long as you're still eating the recommended number of calories per day, then you can ride through this. Have a glass of water, find a good book or take a bath, and remember it isn't long until the morning – who said changing a habit is easy the first time? After a few days, your hunger hormones rebalance – so you have less of the hormones that make you feel hungry and more of the hormones that signal you are full. After about one week, people usually have no hunger by bedtime having eaten early, and are even waking up not hungry and finding it can take one or two hours after waking to start feeling interested in food again.

One of the best ways to stop getting hungry later in the evening is to have around 20g of protein in your evening meal. You could do this for the first week of the 10-Hour Diet to help avoid hunger pangs later in the evening. I have listed common useful foods and quantities of protein within them in Chapter 7 to give you a rough idea and help you with deciding what to include in your evening meals. You won't have to do this for all three months, as usually the hunger pangs last the first week only. But it's a good tool to help if you need it.

10-HOUR DIET SUCCESS

Here is a lady I recently worked with in my clinic whose story we are sharing here:

This female was overweight and said she had an addiction

to sugar. She was suffering inflammation in her back and shoulders and had been prescribed steroids, which had made her put on additional weight. Her old diet started with tea with milk at 7am and ended with eating a little dark chocolate at 10pm before bed. When she switched to having a flax/kefir/berry shake for breakfast instead of a brioche bun and honey with soy milk, having her main meal at lunchtime and a light supper at 6pm, the weight started to come off quite quickly. Stopping eating at 6pm automatically stopped the big G&T, followed by a big meal, followed by treats, that she used to have. She said eating the main meal earlier in the day meant she didn't feel hungry or deprived in the evenings.

Over three months she went from 77kg to 68kg (a loss of over a stone, or more than 19 pounds), was in less pain and was working with her doctor on reducing her steroid prescription for the inflammation. She was also able to come off statins.

Snacks or no snacks?

Some people like to have two meals and one snack. If you need a snack slot, get a piece of fresh fruit or/and a handful of mixed nuts into your diet – all the science shows the chemicals in the colours and fibre in fruit and nuts improve health. Think about what you'll have at the ready for a snack, and where in the day it can go.

Eating non-stop or multiple times a day isn't good for insulin and weight (see Chapter 2), or your bank balance, or digestion, so try to keep your eating events to two or three a day if you can.

For example, I have met people who practise the 10-Hour Diet while working from home. They eat a filling cooked breakfast at 8am; have a piece of fruit such as an apple and a handful of mixed nuts in the middle of the day (which they say saves them time with food prep or going out to find food), and eat dinner at 5.30pm, finishing at 6pm at home. Their eating window is 8am–6pm. They often sling dinner in the oven around 4pm or 4.30pm while working at home (e.g. they bake a sweet potato, which can be served with black beans from a tin and lots of grated cheddar). (See Chapter 6 for more quick Working From Home (WFH) meal ideas which can cook themselves while you work or do other things.)

Final preparations

What to have ready for your fast

- Water, still (habitually) or sparkling (for more special occasions, so you have something interesting when socialising)
- Black coffee/black tea (if you aren't too stressed)
- Green tea – it has a little caffeine to get you started and an amino acid called L-theanine to simultaneously calm you down*

- White tea – contains some caffeine, tastes delicious without milk or sugar and has a mild taste
- Certain herbal teas (see Chapter 8)
- Non calorific drinks – such as iced herbal teas or warm herbal teas
- Your prescription medications

*Coffee has more caffeine than black tea, black tea has more than green tea, green tea has more than white tea. Make your choice according to what you can handle.

Examples of what to avoid during your fast

- Any kind of milks or sugar in your teas and coffees
- Zero-calorie fizzy drinks – the artificial sweeteners in these could make you more hungry (for more on this, see box below)
- Wine, beers or any alcohol
- Supplements
- Children's leftovers, nibbles of food left about
- Sips and bites of other people's snacks
- Coconut water/green juice/kombucha etc. (just because they are deemed 'healthy' or you are having a 'small' portion, doesn't mean they don't count!)

A NOTE ON ZERO-CALORIE DRINKS WITH ARTIFICIAL SWEETENERS

Artificial sweeteners such as aspartame and sucralose are a controversial topic in the research world, where suspicions continue that they may make you more hungry, so put you at risk of weight gain and type 2 diabetes. They have been shown to disrupt gut bacteria (the microbiome) in animal studies. This disruption (known as 'dysbiosis') could lead to feeling hungry continually. This is why avoiding them is a precautionary practice if your goal is weight loss and long-term health.

CAFFEINATED HOT DRINKS – THE PROS AND CONS

Potential negatives:

1. They can trigger anxiety when drunk on an empty stomach.
2. They can drive up stress hormone cortisol (not a good idea if you are already very stressed), which could promote storage of fat around the middle of the body.
3. They can impact sleep – in some sensitive people caffeine stays in the bloodstream for up to 40 hours, depending on whether you are a fast or slow metaboliser! Definitely don't drink it past midday.

4. Caffeine is a laxative – weigh up if you need that help or not.

Potential positives:

1. They can give you a bit of get-up-and-go in the morning until you open your eating window and make the fast easier to prolong later into the morning.
2. They contain polyphenols – the deep dark colours that fight cancer – although you can also get these from many fruit and vegetables.
3. Can improve autophagy – the process where the body slings out old cells and repairs organs (the remodelling effect). The polyphenols (plant chemicals in the colour) rather than the caffeine are the potent substance here.

Look at these two lists and make a cost/benefit calculation. Are you someone who gets a fast heart rate/slightly shaky/more anxious drinking black coffee on an empty stomach?

In my clinic I meet a lot of highly-stressed high-flyers. Black coffee can cause extra stress for some of them and I recommend herbal teas instead such as ginger tea. Even green tea is a better option than coffee for some people. You get the caffeine boostas well as an amino acid called L-theanine, which reduces anxiety and relaxes the brain.

It's important with fasting to hit the sweet spot – where you rev up the body's healing mechanisms without stressing it out. This is where personalisation of this programme is important to make sure you choose the right fit for you.

Now let's go to Chapter 6 for meals that you can get on the table fast to help you nail your timings.

CHAPTER SIX

Real Fast Food

In this section I'll share with you some easy, quick meals I have designed to fit 10-Hour Diet timings, which will set you up well for your day and help you eat earlier, finishing by 8pm at the latest.

I find that the key to eating more of your food earlier in the day is to be able to get food on the table fast. Instead of the usual, ultra-processed Junk Fast Food, however, I want to help you to be able to do that without resorting to food which doesn't earn its place at the table nutritionally. So, these recipes contain meals that are quick, filling *and* good for you.

As we've seen, to gain benefits from the 10-Hour Diet, you only need to concentrate on the timings of your eating, so by all means continue with your usual diet if that's what you decide.

However, if, like many people in my clinic, you want to boost results, then I recommend upgrading some of the content of your diet at the same time as keeping to the 10-hour eating window followed by the 14-hour overnight fast.

FEED YOUR MICROBIOME

We now know that key to health is our microbiome, the trillions of bacteria that live in our digestive system. These bugs in our guts are constantly in cross-talk with our immune system and brain. They also influence our hunger hormones, so it's important to feed the good bugs the right stuff so they thrive and keep these other systems in the body healthy.

When you have your 14-hour overnight fast, these bacteria will proliferate and flourish in a healthy pattern, making you less hungry and your immune system work more peacefully and usefully. Just like, if you were trying to grow a new lawn, you would tell everyone not to walk over it, your gut microbiome also needs a break from food so it has a chance to flourish and grow.

You can also help your microbiome by incorporating a diversity of plants into your diet, as well as specific 'alive' foods, many of which are included in the recipes in this chapter.

By *diversity* I mean including a variety of colour and fibre from vegetables, fruit (fresh or frozen), herbs (fresh or dried) and spices, nuts, seeds, pulses and beans, and extra virgin olive oil. The colour in plants, known as polyphenols, and the texture of them, the fibre, are key to feeding your gut bacteria. So, even if you are eating cheese on toast, follow it with a nice juicy apple for the pectin fibre or a few berries with some live yoghurt (see next point), so you get some polyphenols.

If you like grains, try lots of different ones, instead of sticking to wheat all the time. There are many other tasty, nutritious options, such as spelt, quinoa, black rice and red rice (for those lovely polyphenol colours as well as fibre). To help you train yourself to widen your range of plants in your diet each week, use my Diveristy Challenge worksheet at the end of this book. Here you can record every different plant you eat each week. Try to get between 30 and 60 if you can.

Any time you choose 'alive', rather than 'dead' foods, you've upgraded your diet. Look on dairy labels to see if there are beneficial bacteria in them – on yoghurts, for example, look for ingredients like 'lactobacillus' or 'bifidobacteria'. Or simply look for the word 'live'. Many fermented foods say 'live' and don't list the exact bacteria, which can actually be a good sign, because it means there are too many varied ones from batch to batch to list accurately. When buying cheese, look for the word 'raw' or 'unpasteurised', as these will deliver lots of healthy bacteria into your digestive system. Fermented foods include raw cheeses such as Parmesan, Manchego, Comté, Gruyère, Roquefort, and some Manchegos. You can even buy unpasteurised butter in some supermarkets now. Choose sourdough bread over regular for its beneficial bacteria.

Feeding your microbiome lots of live foods and a diversity of plants, pulses, grains, seeds and nuts can help improve your digestion and immune system so you become more tolerant of more foods if you have had problems in the past.

Other goodies to look out for include kombucha (a sparkling fermented tea), kefir (like a fizzy drinking yoghurt) and kimchi (Asian fermented vegetables) or sauerkraut (Eastern European fermented tangy cabbage), which can likely be found in the fridge section of your supermarket or health food store. If they are sitting on a shelf elsewhere at ambient temperature, this indicates that these are likely 'dead' food. Look for the word 'fermented' on labels, which means they contain bacteria, which is different to 'pickled', which just means the food has been preserved in vinegar (and is 'dead').

The following types of meals will be the most useful for your 10-Hour Diet, and some have the added benefit of being easily portable – handy if you're eating away from home or are on the go.

- **High teas** – High tea is a brilliant invention. It's basically a meal you can get on the table quickly with minimal cooking. I hope to help it make a comeback in our busy lives. In Germany, many people only have one cooked meal of the day – usually at lunch – and their *abendbrot* (literal translation: 'evening bread') is their equivalent of high tea at around 6pm. It's super-convenient and a perfect fit for the 10-Hour Diet. So, if you've already had a hot lunch, you don't have to do a big cook when you get home. You can get lots of plant variety in alongside your cheese, eggs, cold cuts etc., with vegetables from a jar or tin, and side salads or soups. Although my high teas are designed for the last meal of the day, you could easily switch them for lunch. There is lots of flexibility and many are just self-assembly jobs.

- **Quick bowls** – These are pretty one-bowl dishes for one or two people which can be assembled quickly at home for lunches or suppers.
- **Power shakes** – You'll need some emergency shake recipes as meal replacements for breakfast, lunch, snack or supper. These get lots of nutrition into you at high speed if you don't have time to prepare anything more complex. You'll need a blender to prepare most of them.
- **Breakfasts** – Who says breakfast has to be eaten at breakfast? Fine if you are conventional, but all round the world people eat a variety of meals, from lentil soup to rice and curry for breakfast, so have whatever you love. If you want leftovers splashed in chilli sauce, go for it. Or if you like traditional breakfast options like porridge or fry-ups, slot them into any mealtime you fancy. I sometimes crave an açai bowl (recipe below) full of polyphenols. It is one of my favourite quick evening suppers if I've already had a hot meal at lunch.
- **Hearty hot meals** – These are the roasts with all the trimmings and traybakes you can produce for larger numbers of people and lovely weekend

lunches or family evening meals. Many are simply shop-assemble-oven jobs. They also yield great leftovers.

- **Drinks** – You'll need these both to have in your eating window and also to help power your fast.

High Tea

Lemon + dill creamy salmon on toast

THIS MIXTURE MAKES ENOUGH TO COVER 4 SLICES OF TOAST

200g cream cheese
50g smoked salmon
¼ tsp dried dill (and an additional sprinkling to garnish)
Large sprinkling of ground black pepper
Juice of one lemon
Handful of washed rocket leaves
1–2 slices sourdough bread of your choice per person
A knob of butter per slice of bread

Whizz the cream cheese, salmon, dill, black pepper and lemon juice in a blender until smooth.

Toast 2 slices of sourdough bread per person.

Spread butter on the bread and let it sink in (yum!) before placing a handful of rocket leaves on top. Then dollop the cream cheese/ salmon mixture on top and sprinkle with a little more dried dill to garnish.

Egg mayo with watercress on spelt crackers

FEEDS 1

2 boiled eggs (you can make these in advance and store in the fridge)
A dollop of good-quality mayonnaise – get one with olive oil if you can
2 spelt crackers (I use Dr Karg's)
Sea salt
A punnet of watercress

Boil your eggs in water – about 8–10 minutes, so both the white and yolk become set. Either make in advance or, if not, cool them down by running cold water on the eggshells after taking them out of the boiling water. Then peel off the shells and mash the eggs in a bowl with the mayo and sea salt.

Spread the egg mixture on the crackers and sprinkle fresh-cut watercress on top to serve.

Sardines on toast with roasted red peppers

FEEDS 1

1 slice of bread of your choice
1 knob of butter
120g tin of sardines in olive oil
A few strips of roasted red peppers in olive oil (you can buy these in jars and they are great to have stored in your fridge)
Ground black pepper

Toast your bread and spread it with butter. Break up the sardines with a fork on the toast and spread around a little, including all the nutritious bones, and lay strips of red pepper on top.

Serve at once with ground pepper generously sprinkled on top.

Baked beans on toast with Worcestershire sauce and cheddar

FEEDS 2

Everyone in the UK knows how to assemble this high-tea meal, but for any international readers, here goes . . .

400g tin of baked beans
Knob of butter per person
Thick slice of sourdough bread, toasted, per person
Splash of Worcestershire sauce
Handful of grated extra mature cheddar cheese

Heat the beans through in a saucepan.

Toast your bread and then butter it.

Put on a plate, and then pour your beans on top of the buttered toast.

Splash a little Worcestershire sauce on top (it's a delicious salty, fermented condiment if you're not familiar with it . . .)

Scatter a handful of grated extra mature cheese on top (I go for extra mature as the flavour is so much more tangy, and it helps to spice up the somewhat bland beans).

Cheese on toast with gherkins

FEEDS 1

I love how you can take a dish like cheese on toast and make it more healthy by choosing better-quality ingredients. So, instead of using ultra-processed regular white sliced bread (which contains all sorts of preservatives and emulsifiers), pick a bread with as many different nuts, seeds and fibre, such as flax or psyllium husk, and different types of grains in them as you can find. Then swap the processed cheese (e.g. the ones with colourings in them) for a raw, unpasteruised cheese such as Manchego or Gruyère. I'm a fan of keeping fermented live gherkins in the fridge for dishes like this, as they are a healthy form of vegetable containing probiotic bacteria if you don't have any fresh vegetables to hand.

1–2 slices of bread (try to find one with lots of different grains and nuts and seeds in it)
Knob of butter per slice of bread
75g raw unpasteurised cheese such as Manchego or Gruyère per slice of bread
A couple of sliced fermented gherkins per slice of toast (you could use the ones pickled in vinegar for flavour and fibre if you can't find the more nutritious fermented probiotic ones)

Lightly toast your bread and spread with butter.

Arrange the cheese in slices on top of the toast and place under the grill section of your oven if you have one. Wait for the cheese to bubble – watch closely as the length of time (just a couple of minutes in some cases) will depend on the grill you are using and can easily burn.

Take out, slice your gherkins on top and enjoy.

Note: If you have a sandwich toaster, you could put the cheese and gherkins between two slices of buttered bread and make it in there if you prefer to have a sealed toasted sandwich.

Rarebit with Gruyère and smoked chipotle sauerkraut

FEEDS 1

For those of you who like your cheese tangy and spiced up, this is for you. I love forking unpasteurised sauerkraut on top of a high-tea dish like this. The cabbage contains vitamin C as well as healthy probiotic bacteria. I wrote this recipe using one of my favourite sauerkrauts – a chipotle one from the Cultured Collective – but you could use any fresh live type purchased from the fridge section of supermarkets, health food stores or online.

2 slices of sourdough bread
75g Gruyère cheese, grated
1 tbsp French mustard
1 tbsp Worcestershire sauce
4 tbsp sauerkraut (any will do, smoked chipotle flavour is delicious if you can get it)

Lightly toast your bread.

Mash the cheese, mustard and Worcestershire sauce together in bowl with a fork.

Spread the cheese mixture on top of the toasted bread and place under the grill. Toast for about five minutes or until the cheese mixture starts to melt and blister.

Top with sauerkraut and enjoy!

Boiled eggs with soldiers

FEEDS 1

This is simplicity at its best! You can make sure you get some fibre with this meal by following it with a nice juicy apple (for some pectin), a

Vitamin C-rich kiwi or a satsuma. For international readers, 'soldiers' are what we in the UK call long strips of toast – the ideal shape for kids (and adults!) to dunk into the egg yolk.

2 boiled eggs

2 slices of bread (vary this, but a white sourdough loaf would be perfect)

Knob of butter per slice of bread

A pinch of sea salt (I like flaky Maldon for the texture)

Put your eggs in boiling water and let them simmer for 6 minutes and remove. You want the egg white to be hard and the egg yolk to be runny.

Put in egg cups with the toasted, buttered bread cut into strips about 2cm wide on the side.

Break off the top quarter of the egg and sprinkle in the sea salt, then dip your toast into the runny egg and eat the egg up alongside dunking the toast.

Beetroot and lemon humus on warm pitta

MAKES ABOUT 6 GENEROUS SERVINGS AND KEEPS WELL IN THE FRIDGE FOR 2–3 DAYS.

4 medium-size beetroots (you can buy these ready cooked from the supermarket)

400g tin of ready cooked chickpeas

1 tbsp tahini (a paste made from sesame seeds and usually found in the 'World' aisle or 'Free From' sections of supermarkets)

Juice of 2 lemons

5 tbsp extra virgin olive oil

½ tsp sea salt flakes

A pinch of ground pepper
A piece of warmed pitta bread per person

Put all the ingredients (except the pitta bread) in a powerful blender and pulse until smooth.

Spoon out into a big sharing bowl and eat spread on warmed pitta bread.

Coronation chicken with pomegranate

FEEDS 2

2 tbsp extra virgin olive oil
1 onion, peeled and finely chopped
3 sticks of celery, finely chopped
1 tsp turmeric
1 tsp ground cumin
2 handfuls of cold chicken (picked off a leftover roast chicken or from 2 chicken legs)
1 jalapeño chilli from a jar, chopped
240ml (or one American cup) fermented milk kefir
Juice of half a lime
Handful of chopped fresh coriander
Handful of pomegranate seeds
Pinch of sea salt
1 little gem lettuce

Heat the oil gently in a pan and add the onion, celery, turmeric and cumin. Stir on and off for 8–10 minutes until the onions are translucent and starting to brown. Remove from heat and allow to cool down.

Combine the onion mixture with the chicken in a bowl and add the jalapeño chilli.

Pour in the kefir and lime juice and stir in the coriander, then sprinkle the pomegranate seeds and a little sea salt on top to serve.

Leave the mixture in the fridge until needed or serve straight away, scooped onto several little gem lettuce leaves.

Quick Bowls

Crispy tofu with miso and broccolini

FEEDS 1

150g organic silken tofu
1 tbsp cornflour
Sprinkling of sea salt
4 tbsp extra virgin olive oil
240ml (or one American cup) chicken or vegetable stock
1 tsp garlic paste*
1 tsp ginger paste*
60g rice noodles
A handful of broccolini stems and heads
1 tsp miso paste
Splash of soy sauce
A handful of sliced spring onions
1 fresh red chilli, sliced and chopped into small pieces
1 tbsp of kimchi, to serve (optional)

Cut the tofu into cubes and blot them gently with kitchen roll.

Put the flour on a plate and mix in a sprinkling of sea salt.

Dip each piece of tofu in the flour, so all sides are covered.

Heat the oil on a medium heat (you could do this in a wok if you have one, although a frying pan would work too) and sauté the cubes of flour-covered tofu until they are slightly crispy on the outside.

Take out the tofu cubes with a slotted spoon and place on a piece of kitchen paper while you make the rest of the meal.

Add your garlic and ginger pastes to the remaining oil in the wok/frying pan. Stir on a low heat for a couple of minutes.

Add the stock and gently heat until the broth boils, then turn down the heat to simmer and add the rice noodles. Let them cook for two minutes.

Now add the broccolini (you could cut the stems in half if they're too long to fit in the wok or pan) and simmer in the stock for about a minute (the broccolini is barely blanched in the liquid and will be served crunchy).

Pour the mixture into a large serving bowl. Tip the tofu cubes on stop. Add a small teaspoon of miso paste (which you can mix in as you eat) and a little dash of soy sauce.

Throw your raw spring onions and chilli on top along with the kimchi to serve.

*Garlic paste and ginger paste are becoming more available in supermarkets, usually in the 'World' section alongside foods for Indian meal ingredients. After opening them, you can keep them in your fridge and use as short cuts when you haven't got much time for peeling and chopping garlic and ginger or don't have any fresh at home.

Jacket potato, black beans and avocado with chipotle

FEEDS 1

1 large Maris Piper, King Edward or Cyprus potato (any white potato could be used, but these varieties are particularly tasty)

A knob of butter

200g tin black beans in chilli sauce

1 tbsp chipotle sauce (this Mexican chilli sauce has a lovely smoky flavour)

A dollop of Greek yoghurt

Half an avocado (store the other half mashed in the fridge with a squeeze of lime to stop discolouration and have on toast next meal)

A sprinkling of sea salt

Juice of half a lime

Wash your potato to get any dirt off the skin, stab 3–4 times with a knife (this stops the skin bursting when cooking) and place in the oven on 200°C degrees for 45 mins to an hour, or until the potato is cooked through and the outside is crispy (time will vary depending on the size of the potato).

Heat the beans in a saucepan on a medium heat for about 2–3 minutes.

Cut the avocado half into slices.

Mix the yoghurt and chipotle together in a small bowl.

To serve, cut the potato in half and top with the butter, beans and then the yoghurt chipotle. Arrange the avocado around the outside, with a little lime juice squeezed on and a pinch of sea salt on top.

Waldorf salad and smoked mackerel

FEEDS 2

1 apple, cored and cut into small cubes

2 tbsp walnut pieces

2 sticks of celery, topped and tailed, cut into pieces about 1cm thick

2 tbsp plain live yoghurt

2 tbsp mayonnaise

1 tbsp horseradish sauce

A sprinkling of sea salt

Pinch of ground pepper

2 fillets of smoked mackerel (you can buy these ready made in the fridge section of supermarkets)

Combine the apple, walnuts and celery in a bowl.

In a cup, mix the yoghurt, mayonnaise, horseradish sauce, salt and pepper.

Pour the yoghurt mix on top of the apple mix and stir through.

Scatter a few pieces of smoked mackerel on top and enjoy.

Build a Bowl

I first developed a table like this (see page 90) for a lady I worked with a few years ago. She did not enjoy cooking. She had spent decades counting calories and eating low-fat processed convenience foods and had a ring around the middle of her body which she was very frustrated about and which would not go away, despite all her dieting. She came to me about her high blood pressure, which she and her doctor had tried to reduce using medications, but the side effects of the drugs were too much for her to bear.

She was motivated to change her eating, but told me she didn't know how to cook. I realised she *did* know how to shop, even if she lacked cooking experience, and so that's when I decided to write a table similar to this for her. I remember the picture of the inside of her fridge she sent me after her first shop – teeming with natural colour from top to bottom! It's all about getting bags of salads into your fridge, lots of the right jars and tins into the house, and learning how to do a self-assembly job on a meal.

After about three months, she lost the extra weight around the middle of her body, her blood pressure came down to normal levels, and she has been able to stay off blood pressure medications ever since.

To use the table, pick one food from each column, and mix and match to create a meal full of interesting, delicious variety which is easy to compile: protein and fats to fill you up, colour to get your natural plant food count up, and fermented foods to get lots of live natural food into you. The sauces are there to make your bowl tasty as well as healthy.

PROTEIN	GOOD FATS	PLANTS
A tin of salmon with a squeeze of lemon juice and ground black pepper	A handful of chopped walnuts	A large handful of mixed salad leaves and a couple of artichokes from a jar
A piece of grass-fed steak with a drizzle of squeezed lime and pinch of sea salt	A handful of chopped Brazil nuts	A large handful of rocket leaves and a handful of chopped coriander
Tinned tuna in olive oil with squeezed lime, chopped coriander and chopped jalapeño peppers from a jar	A tablespoon of roasted pine nuts	A large handful of spinach leaves, a few olives from a jar and a large spoonful of cooked quinoa
Half a tin of chickpeas sautéed in a chopped clove of garlic, one red onion (diced), a little sea salt and some chopped chorizo	A handful of chopped almonds	A sliced yellow pepper, cored, with a couple of juicy ripe tomatoes (sliced)
Half a tin of green lentils with a spoonful of sunblushed tomatoes, a small red onion (diced, raw) and a pinch of sea salt	A handful of pumpkin seeds heated in a pan with a pinch of sea salt and dried chilli flakes for flavour (or just regular ones)	A large handful of watercress leaves and a handful of pomegranate seeds
Beetroot and lemon humus (see recipe in this chapter on page 83)	A drizzle of extra virgin olive oil	A handful of lamb's lettuce leaves, a handful of chopped fresh parsley and a stick of chopped celery
A fillet of smoked mackerel	An avocado sliced with lemon juice and ground pepper on top	Two chicories (white or purple ones, chopped), a ready-cooked beetroot (sliced) and a tangerine or orange (peeled and sliced)

FERMENTS	SAUCES
A spoonful of live white cabbage sauerkraut from a jar – delicious forked through green leaves!	3 tbsp kefir, 1 tbsp olive oil, half a squeezed lemon, handful of chopped chives and a pinch of sea salt
A spoonful of red cabbage sauerkraut from a jar	3 tbsp live yoghurt mixed with 1 tsp chipotle sauce
A few sliced fermented gherkins	1 tsp raw honey, 1 tsp mustard and 2 tbsp olive oil dressing mixed with 2 tbsp live yoghurt
Shavings of Parmesan cheese	A large glug of Catalan ketchup (see page 92 for recipe)
Shavings of Gruyère cheese	A large glug of pesto (from a jar) mixed with 2 tbsp extra virgin olive oil (to make it pourable)
Spoonful of live fermented veg	1 tsp tahini mixed with 3 tbsp live yoghurt, half a squeezed lemon and a pinch of sea salt
Spoonful of fermented jalapeño peppers (drizzle the juice from the jar over the salad too – it'll taste delicious)	Vinaigrette dressing made from 2 tbsp olive oil, 1 tbsp red wine vinegar, 1 tsp Dijon mustard and a pinch of sea salt

Catalan Ketchup

This ketchup keeps in a container in the fridge for 2–3 days. It goes well with grilled vegetables, meat or fish and can also be drizzled over whatever you put in your Build a Bowl.

2 red peppers in olive oil from a jar
1 medium tomato
1 clove of garlic, peeled
2 jalapeño peppers from a jar
1 tsp smoked paprika
A glug of extra virgin olive oil
1 large tbsp ground almonds

Put the ingredients in a blender and pulse until smooth.

Power Shakes

These are designed to give you a quick nutritious breakfast, portable meal or planned snack.

Flax and blueberry shake

200ml organic unsweetened soya milk
1 heaped tbsp ground flaxseeds (also known as linseeds)
A handful of frozen blueberries (much cheaper than fresh)
Half a banana

Put all the ingredients in a blender, mix until smooth, and serve.

Chia and passionfruit shake

200ml organic whole milk or organic unsweetened soya milk
Flesh of 2 passionfruits
1 banana
1 tbsp chia seeds

Put all the ingredients in a blender, mix until smooth, and serve.

Chocolate milkshake

200ml organic unsweetened soya milk
1 tsp cacao powder
1 tbsp ground flaxseeds (also known as linseeds)
1 ice cube
1 banana (optional)

I've designed this one for those of you who don't have a blender. Just put the powdered cacao and flaxseed into a glass with the soya milk and stir. Add ice if you fancy it. If you do have a blender, then whizz all the ingredients up and add a banana, which will sweeten it.

Chia and cherry pot

240ml (or one American cup) kefir (cow's or goat's)
A handful of frozen black cherries
¼ cup (35g) chia seeds
A swirl of maple syrup to serve (optional)

Put all the ingredients in a blender, mix until smooth, and serve. This one is eaten with a spoon!

Note: in recent times nut milks have become popular, but many are nutritionally inferior to animal milk and much more expensive. Pick whichever suits your stomach and wallet best.

If you'd like to substitute animal milk, I often use soya milk nowadays as the protein content is reasonably high, so it makes you feel full for longer than some other nut milks, such as almond or hazelnut. Pick unsweetened and organic if possible (to avoid unnecessary sugar and the concerns about regular soya milks, which are often genetically modified).

High-protein Shakes

The following two shakes are useful breakfasts to have after working out or could be helpful meal replacement options in the evening, as they each contain around 20g of protein, which is about the amount that will keep you feeling full for several hours. They use 100% real food, too – no processed protein powders involved.

Super kefir and kiwi shake

This shake may be useful after exercise, but you could have it at any mealtime you like. The coconut water contains electrolytes, the important micro-minerals for your nervous system, which you lose when you sweat. The matcha powder contains antioxidants to counteract muscle damage, and kiwis are high in vitamin C – important for the immune system and healthy connective tissue in the body.

The kefir, soya milk and flax make this shake high in protein (about 20g), which will help you build muscle, repair sore tissue and feel full.

125ml coconut water
1 tsp matcha powder
2 kiwis, peeled
¼ cup (35g) flaxseeds
240ml (or one American cup) milk kefir
100ml soya milk (this helps thin the shake, and adds further protein)

Put all the ingredients in a blender, mix until smooth, and serve.

Soya and seed shake

The soya milk and seed/nut mix deliver 17g protein, while cacao powder and raspberries are powerful polyphenol antioxidants. The banana sweetens the shake and replaces electrolytes.

240ml (one American cup) soya milk
35g/¼ cup mixed ground nuts and seeds*
A handful of frozen or fresh raspberries
Half a banana
1 tbsp cacao powder

Put all the ingredients in a blender, mix until smooth, and serve.

*All supermarkets, from budget to upmarket, are now selling interesting mixes of ground nuts. Brazil nuts, flax and almonds, or sunflower, pumpkin and sesame are mixes that come to mind. There are lots of different ones out there – rotate different mixes to increase the variety of foods you eat each day.

Breakfasts

Bircher muesli

MAKES ABOUT 3 SERVINGS

125g/1 ⅓ cup oats
2 squeezed oranges
400ml Greek yoghurt or fermented milk kefir
1 tbsp ground flaxseeds
1 tbsp chopped walnuts
1 apple, cored and grated
Handful of pomegranate seeds (optional)
Splash of apple juice (optional)

Combine all the ingredients in a bowl, stir, and place, covered overnight, in your fridge until you want to spoon out a serving.

This will keep well in the fridge for 2–3 days, but if the mixture is a bit stiff (which can happen if you use thick Greek yoghurt instead of kefir, which is a bit thinner), then stir in a splash of apple juice.

Açai bowl

SERVES 1

You could eat this for breakfast, lunch or supper – it's totally interchangeable.

100g açaí frozen purée pouch (available in supermarkets as well as health food stores nowadays)
Half a banana
Splash of nut or animal milk such as cow's or goat's

Dollop of Greek yoghurt
1 tsp peanut butter
Handful of chopped walnuts
Handful of a low-sugar granola
Sprinkling of cacao nibs
1 kiwi, peeled and sliced

Put the contents of the açai pouch (still frozen) in a powerful blender with half a banana to sweeten it and a splash of milk of your choice to loosen the mixture into a nice purple slush!

Pour the slush into a large bowl and get artistic – a dollop of yoghurt, peanut butter, and then sprinkle your walnuts, granola, cacao nibs and a row of sliced kiwi on top to serve.

Raspberry and pistachio silky porridge

SERVES 1

I once worked with a couple of five-star hotel chefs and witnessed a vehement exchange about how many minutes you should boil your porridge to get it to the loveliest consistency. Their eventual answer was 40 minutes! It must be 'silky' in texture, they said. Once you've tried porridge stewed into a silky consistency, nothing else will do. You could boil your oats with water in a microwave for a couple of minutes (thumbs down sign), or you could stew it like they do for 40 (thumbs up sign). If you are trying to delay breakfast, to elongate your fast, maybe 40 minutes will do you just fine! I promise the first mouthful when you are really hungry and ready to open your 10-hour eating slot will be worth it! I sometimes make this in my rice cooker for 40 minutes as it's easier to clean than a saucepan.

30g/⅓ cup oats per person

240ml/1 cup water (yes, water, because milk can curdle in that amount of time. You can always add a splash of milk on serving if you like the taste)

A teeny pinch of sea salt

A scattering of chopped pistachios (expensive but delicious; you only need a tablespoon and this will make it a more filling meal)

Dollop of raspberry jam (the taste of raspberry and pistachio is a delicious combo)

Put the oats, water and pinch of sea salt in a saucepan, bring to the boil, lower the heat and let stew with a tilted lid on (allowing a little steam out as it cooks) for 40 minutes. If you have a slow cooker or rice cooker, you could follow instructions on those.

When ready, turn off the heat.

Serve in a bowl with the pistachios, raspberry jam and a splash of milk on top.

Antioxidant English breakfast

SERVES 2

English breakfasts get such a bad press. With a range of tasty plants in there – tomatoes, mushrooms, courgette, black beans and rocket, for example – you can get lots of antioxidants to counterbalance the nitrates in the bacon (which may be carcinogenic in large quantities in a diet with little veg to counteract them).

4 slices smoked streaky bacon or pancetta

Splash of extra virgin olive oil (high polyphenol count helps protect this oil from damage when heated)

Large handful of cherry tomatoes, halved

Handful per person of any type of mushrooms you fancy, sliced
1 small courgette, topped and tailed
Sprinkle of sea salt and ground pepper
2 whisked eggs
200g black beans in chilli sauce from a tin (I like Biona)
Handful of washed rocket salad, to serve (optional)

Dry-fry the bacon in a frying pan on a medium heat on the hob until crispy (or however you like it!), then remove to a plate and put in your oven on a low heat to keep warm while you cook the rest of the breakfast.

Add a splash of extra virgin olive oil to the pan if needed alongside the remaining fat in the pan from the bacon.

Sauté the cherry tomatoes on one side of the pan and the mushrooms on the other until both are soft and slightly shrunken (add a little more oil if needed). Keep these warm alongside the bacon in the oven.

Grate the courgette and then sauté in the pan using any oil still there, or add a small drop more if needed. Stir for a minute or two until cooked through. Sprinkle with a little salt and pepper.

Add the whisked eggs to the courgette and stir around until they start to set, then remove from the heat. Season to taste.

Warm your beans in a microwave or a saucepan for a couple of minutes.

Add the eggs and beans to the plate from the oven with all the other ingredients and enjoy.

Hearty Hot Meals

Slow-roasted chicken with apple

SERVES 4

1 medium-size chicken
1 apple
2 tbsp extra virgin olive oil
1 tsp sea salt
1 tsp dried oregano
The zest of a lemon, finely grated
2 garlic cloves, peeled and crushed

Unwrap the chicken, cut off any elastic bands and discard the innards should there be any. Place the chicken on a baking tray and put a whole apple inside the cavity of the chicken – no need to peel or core it. This means that the apple will bake as the chicken is cooked and ooze sweet juice into the bird, infusing it with taste and stopping it becoming dry.

Pour the olive oil into a cup and stir in the salt, oregano, lemon peel and garlic.

Pour this mixture onto the bird and massage it into the skin, making sure not to miss the legs, wings and underneath.

Put the chicken in an oven heated to 150°C/300°F and cook for 2 hours. Yes – you read that right. This is cooking super slow, and with the above measures the chicken should come out juicy inside and crispy on top.

Take out of the oven about 15 minutes before serving, put a sheet of tin foil on top to keep it warm, and leave the bird to 'relax' – this move really helps the meat to be tender and fall off the bone.

Carve the joint into pieces and serve, spooning the juices from the pan over each serving of meat (which means you don't have to worry about making gravy).

Mustard glazed gammon

SERVES 4 IF SERVED WITH LOTS OF VEGETABLES

750g piece of smoked gammon
100g French mustard
1 tbsp demerara sugar
1 cup/¼ litre of apple juice

Cut the hard rind off the top of the gammon, leaving the white fleshier fat exposed underneath. With a sharp knife, score the fat to make a crisscross pattern (this will create little lines to suck up the mustard and sugar and make a nice crust in the oven).

Smear mustard and sugar all over, especially pressing into the fatty side.

Get a large piece of tin foil and lay out in a roasting tray so that it cradles the whole pan. Put the gammon in the tray, pour in the apple juice and scrunch the tin foil up at the top so the gammon is totally enveloped, sitting in a puddle of apple juice, which will diffuse into the meat as it cooks.

Put in the oven on 160°C/320°F for 1 hour.

Once an hour has passed, undo the tin foil, fold back to the edges and turn the oven up to 225°C/435°F, making sure the fatty side is facing up. Cook for 15 minutes to crisp up the fat.

Take out of the oven and let the meat stand for a few minutes to 'rest', which I find makes it more tender.

Cut into slices and pour a bit of the salty mustardy apple juice over each portion.

Note: It is important to check that the meat is fully cooked all the way through – eating raw pork is not safe.

Sides with your roasts

You can make any of these sides with any of the meat cuts above:

The world's best crispy roast potatoes

750g Maris Piper, King Edward's or Cyprus potatoes (or any variety that has a specialist name and isn't just called 'white potatoes', which are the ones in supermarkets with hardly any flavour)

Unsalted real butter (there are lots of brands of regular butter – just make sure it isn't one that has been mixed with any cheap industrial fillers, which are found in lots of the ready-to-spread soft butters)

Sea salt

Lots of ground black pepper

Peel the potatoes and cut into quarters.

Put them in a saucepan with a teaspoon of sea salt and cover with water. Wait until the water boils, then reduce heat to simmer.

Simmer the potatoes for at least 10 minutes and drain them when they are soft on the outside but still a bit firm inside (you can test with a fork), but not falling apart.

Now, this is the important bit: after draining, put the potatoes back in the saucepan, put the butter on top, put the lid on, and shake the pot until the potatoes get covered in the butter. This will also cause the outside of the potatoes to become fluffy and rough-edged, which is crucial for getting a really crisp potato ...

Put the potatoes on a baking tray and sprinkle with sea salt and lots of ground black pepper. Cook in an oven at 220°C/425°F for about half an hour until the edges are all crispy.

Serve at once. (You might like to try to calm the atmosphere of guests and family with a glass of wine – tempers can run high competing for the crispiest spuds!)

The easiest vegetable tray bake

For this recipe, I go to the supermarket and buy one of those packs designed for making stews, found in the fruit and veg aisle. They cost next to nothing and come with an onion, a leek and a few pieces of root vegetables such as a swede, carrot, parsnip etc.

Root vegetable mix
4 tbsp extra virgin olive oil
A sprinkling of sea salt and a generous grinding of black pepper

Peel and quarter the onion.

Top and tail the leek and cut into slices about 3cm thick.

Peel the root vegetables and cut into cubes.

Scatter all the vegetables over a large baking tray and drizzle with the olive oil and seasonings.

Cook at 200°C/390°F for about 40 minutes, taking it out half way through to give everything a shake.

When the vegetables are slightly crispy and soft in the middle (you can test with a fork), you are ready to serve.

Carrot, sweet potato and crispy leek chip mix

2 carrots
1 large sweet potato
1 large leek
4 tbsp extra virgin olive oil
A sprinkling of sea salt and lots of ground black pepper

Wash the leek and cut off the hard end. Cut into three and then slice each piece lengthways.

Wash the carrots, cut off the hard ends and cut into the shape of chips.

Peel the sweet potato and cut into the shape of chips.

Place all the veg on a baking tray, drizzle in olive oil, then sprinkle with sea salt and ground black pepper.

Place in an oven and bake on 200°C/390°F for 30–40 minutes until the orange veg is cooked through and the leeks are a little crispy.

Tray Bakes

Chorizo, fennel, sweet potato, red onions and butter beans

SERVES 4

Rich and hearty for a cold winter night, this tray bake is quick to prepare and you can get on with other things while it cooks.

6 large chorizo sausages (about 400g in total) cut into large chunks (about 4 pieces per sausage)
1 fennel, topped and tailed, cut into eighths

1 sweet potato, peeled and cut into chips

1 white sweet onion (regular yellow onions will do if you can't find the sweet white Spanish ones), peeled and cut into eighths

400g tin of butter beans

Sprinkling of smoked paprika

Scattering of sea salt and ground black pepper

Drizzle of extra virgin olive oil

Spread out the chorizo, fennel, sweet potato, onion and beans on a large baking tray, season with the paprika, salt and pepper, and drizzle with olive oil. Place in the oven for 40 minutes on 200°C/390°F. The sweet potatoes should be cooked through and the fennel soft, all oozing with orange-coloured paprika oil from the chorizo.

Serve in individual bowls. (You'll need a spoon as well as a knife and fork to catch all the sauce!)

Harissa potato with halloumi and green olives

SERVES 2

1 large potato, skin on, washed and cut into small cubes

1 tbsp harissa paste

1 red pepper, cored and cut into thin slices

1 large red onion, peeled and cut into eighths

10 large pitted green olives, halved

6 cloves of garlic, skin left on to avoid burning (you can push the flesh out with your fork as you eat this dish)

225g halloumi, cut into eight slices

Sprinkling of sumac (this is a Middle Eastern tangy yet mild spice found easily in supermarkets these days)

Sprinkling of sea salt

4 tbsp extra virgin olive oil
Dollop of hummus, to serve (optional)

Put the potato cubes in a bowl, add the harissa and stir through so all the potatoes are nicely coated before scattering them on a large baking tray.

Add the red pepper, onion, olives and garlic, then dot the slices of halloumi around on top of those.

Sprinkle the sumac and sea salt onto the mix and drizzle everything in the pan with the olive oil.

Place in the oven on 225°C/435°F for about 45 minutes or until the potatoes and vegetables are cooked through and the halloumi is a little crispy. (Ten minutes before the end, give the mixture a gentle stir.)

Plate up and include a spoonful of hummus on the side if liked.

Drinks to power your fast

- Iced herbal teas (check they contain one calorie or less – beware as some have much more – see FAQ chapter for more on this) and fizzy water
- Warm herbal teas of your choice (I'm a fan of Wise Owl for the varied options and flavours)
- Caffeinated drinks such as black coffee, black tea, white tea and green tea are all good options in the morning until you break your fast (try not to have these in the afternoon, however, as they could negatively impact your sleep)

- Water infused with fresh herbs e.g. water infused with mint

HOW MUCH PROTEIN DOES A REGULAR PERSON NEED PER DAY?

Multiply your weight in kilos by 0.75g to find how much you need. (Source: Food Standards Agency)

For example, if you are 70kg you would need 52g per day.

Protein at each meal is essential to make us feel full, as it digests more slowly than any other foods. If we are full, we are less likely to graze! We also need it to build skin, tissue, muscle, bone, and our mind. It is the building block of our physical tissues, our hormones (the chemical messengers) and neurotransmitters in the brain that contribute to our mood and help us sleep. It helps weight loss because the body burns up more calories breaking it down than other food groups. We spend energy eating it, a process called thermogenesis. It is much overlooked and often gets lost in the fanfare of other food types, so keep an eye on it.

Stressed individuals may need higher levels of protein. All the hormones in the body, including the stress ones such as adrenaline and cortisol, are made from protein, so you may be getting through lots if you are having a stressful time. Athletes also have higher protein needs.

How Much Protein Is In Which Foods?

This a snapshot of some commonly-eaten protein foods so you can quickly gauge quantities. I feel that highlighting protein in this book is important so that you can include some protein to feel full up throughout your evening until you go to bed. If you feel full after your last meal of the day, you will have a much more comfortable and successful 14-hour overnight fast.

The numbers on the right indicate the amount of protein within the food. Sometimes just adding a handful of seeds to salads or porridge, or throwing some cheese shavings over roast vegetables, can make a big difference to how full you feel after your meal.

Nuts and seeds

QUANTITY	FOOD	PROTEIN CONTENT IN GRAMS
¼ cup/155g	Flaxseeds	8
¼ cup/170g	Chia seeds	5
¼ cup/100g	Almonds	5
¼ cup/135g	Cashews	6
¼ cup/110g	Flax, pumpkin and sesame mix	7

Milk

200ml/¾ cup	Nut milks	2
200ml/¾ cup	Soya milk	6
200ml/¾ cup	Cow's milk	7

Soya

166g/1 cup	Tempeh	31
150g/¾ cup	Silken tofu	11

Beans and pulses (tinned, cooked)

400g	Chickpeas	18
400g	Kidney beans	18
400g	Baked beans	18
400g	Black beans	15
400g	Green lentils	14

Yoghurt, cheese, eggs

200ml/¾ cup	Cow's milk kefir	10
150g/⅗ cup	Greek yoghurt	15
240ml/1 cup	Coconut kefir	3
28g	Parmesan cheese	11
65g	Cheddar cheese	16
100g	Halloumi	22
50g	Goat's cheese	9
1	Egg	7

Fish and seafood

200g	Cod	46
100g/1 cup	Prawns	24
100g	Smoked salmon	18
200g	Smoked haddock	50
100g	Tinned sardines	24

Meats

200g	Chicken breast	54
200g	Duck breast	49
200g	Beef	52
200g	Lamb	50
1 medium slice	Ham	9

Some protein-rich plants

130g/1 cup	Green peas	4
30g/½ cup	Mushrooms	2
180g/1 cup	Quinoa, cooked	8

Shortcuts

Cut up lemons into quarters and keep them in the freezer in bags. You can run them under a hot tap and use them whenever needed. I also pop frozen lemon quarters straight into a glass of water to make it a bit more exciting sometimes.

Frozen foods are getting ever more exciting and varied, and vegetables and fruits from the freezer retain their plant chemicals and fibre. Recent frozen findings I've enjoyed include sweet potato chips, pomegranate seeds and cauliflower hash browns. If you haven't looked at the frozen vegetable and fruit sections of supermarkets for a while, go back and have another look. You may find you have less food wastage, too, buying vegetables or fruits such as berries and herbs frozen rather than fresh. They are also often cheaper than fresh ones.

You can cheer up almost any meal by taking a big dollop of live, plain yoghurt or milk kefir, and stirring a dollop of chipotle paste, or other type of chili sauce of your choice, into it. You can dunk your oven-roasted vegetables into it, or put some in a packed lunchbox with leftover meats, cold poached fish and salads.

Keep tins in your cupboards to get meals on the table quickly when needed. Beans and pulses of all types – from lentils and black beans to butter beans – can help you create a nutritious, filling meal in minutes. You can even stir the lentils or butter beans into a bought soup to make it more filling and bump up the protein content. Tinned fish is another source of quick meals.

Key to making any quick meal interesting is to have good condiments and marinades in your fridge. Cheese can be cheered up with a tasty tomato chutney; any defrosted white fish can be made delicious with some harissa smeared on top of it before grilling. My favourite condiment in recent times is the Turkish dry sweet pepper flakes known as Pul Biber. You can sprinkle these on top of almost any meal to make it look pretty and give it a little kick. Pul Biber can bring flavour to a vegetable as bland as steamed cauliflower if you sprinkle it on top with some lemon juice and sea salt. Yotam Ottolenghi, who is a master of the multi-ingredient dish, uses Pul Biber in his latest cookbook, *Flavour,* and refers to it as Aleppo pepper. Hopefully, as a result, it'll now become more widely available. You don't have to go all far-flung on your spices and condiments, either. I find grinding loads of black pepper onto bland dishes like potatoes or soups made of root vegetables can make them really tasty. Whether you like mustards and pickles with your cheese, horseradish sauce on your smoked mackerel or wasabi in your salad dressing, stock up with some dramatic flavours. It'll make a big difference to home-prepared meals and many contain plant chemicals in the colour or fibre, both of which are good for us.

CHAPTER SEVEN

Frequently Asked Questions

Do I have to change what I eat to see results?

During the 10-hour eating slot you can eat heartily, and it is up to you what you eat. I suggest you don't graze, however, as long gaps between food are more effective for weight loss.

This diet is about working with you on your timings to get great results. The content is up to you. The main point being, by focusing on optimal timing of eating, you can keep your usual diet going and still lose weight. Of course it'll work better if you eat healthier food, but all the studies have been conducted on subjects who did not change *what* they ate – only *when*. And all of them saw results.

That said, try to eat unprocessed food where you can and include lots of different fresh fruit and vegetables in your diet, as everyone benefits from these actions, whether vegetarian or meat eater, pescatarian or vegan etc.

What if I'm already following a diet based on the type of food I eat?

An advantage of this programme is that you can drop your new eating timings into other eating plans if you wish. So, if you already follow a vegan, vegetarian, paleo, ketogenic or Mediterranean diet, for example, you can work the principles of the 10-Hour Diet into the mix.

Can I eat anything I like on this diet and get results?

If you usually eat junk food, you can continue to do this. But if you usually don't eat junk food, this isn't the time to start. In studies, the diet is usually kept the same as before the 10-hour eating habit is introduced. However, many people in my clinical practice use the new timings to upgrade the quality of their diet for extra success (see Chapter 6 for recipe ideas for nutritious meals). Try as much as you can to stick to proper meals (two or three each day) and avoid grazing (e.g. sugary drinks – including tea with sugar – between meals would count as grazing), which is thought to upset many metabolic mechanisms in the body. Have your tea without sugar and milk and you're not snacking. In Germany, black tea is traditionally drunk without milk – it's a bit of English habit, that one. It can taste delicious and feel reviving once you get used to it, so why not give it a try?

Should I limit the amount of food I eat?

Listen to your appetite; eat as much as you need to feel properly full, and then stop. Many people find that their hunger hormones, which signal when they are full or hungry, are more audible after a week of the 10-Hour Diet.

You can lose weight if you eat your usual background diet or improve it, but if you were to double the quantity of your usual diet, you would be very unlikely to see results. The studies have always told participants to continue their usual background diet, and most ended up reducing their daily calorie intake by 20% just by stopping eating by 6pm or 8pm, probably because alcohol and sweet-treat opportunities went down. They also saw benefits to their health markers and experienced less hunger by stopping earlier – no changes to the content of their normal diet involved.

Can I eat or drink anything during the fasting period?

Everything you eat or drink outside the 10 hours (apart from water, certain herbal teas, black tea and coffee) is counted as breaking the fast. So, if you have a cup of tea with a splash of milk at 7am, you have broken the fast with the milk. Or if you have a sip of wine or a handful of somebody else's popcorn at 9pm, you haven't begun fasting yet. Remember that many of the mechanisms that make this diet effective are switched on during the 12–14-hour fasted state, so stay strong! If you eat or drink in this slot, it's unlikely you'll reap all the benefits!

Can I have black tea and coffee?

Technically, yes, for some people these are a helpful tool to get through the early morning without food. But for certain people, black coffee or tea containing caffeine may boost your stress hormone cortisol, making weight loss more difficult if you are having a particularly stressful time. Ask yourself if this is you or not and decide accordingly if you will be drinking black coffee/tea or caffeine-free herbal alternatives during your fast for best results. For some people black coffee and tea work fine, for others herbal teas work better in the morning. Self-experiment.

When should I break my fast in the morning?

You can set your own eating schedule based on what you find easiest to do. For instance, if you are someone who never feels hungry in the morning, skip breakfast and begin your 10-hour eating window later in the morning. For many people, the 10-Hour Diet simply means starting breakfast a little later (or missing it if they aren't a breakfast eater) and bringing supper forward a bit.

How many meals should I have during my 10-hour eating window?

You can choose whether to have two or three meals during your 10-hour eating slot. You can have a planned snack if you need one, but try not to graze.

Some people eat three meals during the week and two meals at weekends, when they get up later. Choose what suits your lifestyle best. Some people have two meals every day and a small snack. Some have two main meals, some people three. The good news is that you can design your eating pattern how you like within your 10-hour slot, as long as you aim to be done by 8pm. Self-experiment to get the right pattern for your body going.

As mentioned in a previous chapter, I'm a big believer in run-in preparation periods to gain confidence and achieve more. Changing habits, in my opinion, is all about mastery and practice. Look in your diary. Think about changing one meal first – e.g. could you skip breakfast and go through to lunchtime on just a black tea, or push breakfast back to mid-morning? Or perhaps you are someone who loves breakfast and lunch, so you might decide to make those your two main meals, and just have something light at 5pm and then stop eating for the rest of the day. You might like to carry one of my shakes with you (see recipes in Chapter 6) as a breakfast or 5pm light meal if you are likely to need a portable, nutritious meal to have while out and about, or to consume quickly if you are a Working From Homer. You may find, having had a decent breakfast and lunch, that you don't need any more food that day, and that the weight comes off easiest for you when you finish eating early.

Should I do early or late TRE?

Often, larks find early TRE gets them best results, whereas late TRE suits owls better, but there isn't enough evidence to be categorical about this, so try both out for yourself.

I personally lose weight if I eat between 8am and 6pm, known as early TRE. This works for me, as I'm at my most productive early in the day. If I eat between 10am and 8pm (late TRE), I don't see the same results.

Of course, this isn't the case for everyone, so give yourself a couple of weeks to practice and discover the timings that work for you practically, that suit your personal physiology and that get you the results you desire. You'll quickly see what events are sabotaging you and you can then think of practical solutions. (See page 43 for a template you can use for this.)

When should I eat my biggest meal to lose weight?

Eating our main meal earlier in the day may yield more weight loss than later for some people. This is because early eating is aligned with our circadian rhythm (the clocks in the body controlled by light and eating, which trigger many mechanisms to work best by day). Many enzymes connected with digestion and metabolism work in a time-of-day-specific way.

The problem with modern-day society is that food is winking at us at all times of the day and night, and we are shoving food into us when the body isn't able to process it properly. This leads to confusion and disorder of many systems – from our hormones and metabolism to heart function.

How much weight will I lose?

People I have worked with tend to lose about a pound a week in weight without going hungry or having to count calories – though for people with a body mass index of over 25 (overweight and obese categories), it tends to be much more.

In TRE studies, with no changes whatsoever to the actual content of their diets, people lose up to 5 per cent of their body weight in four months and at least 3 per cent in three months. In my practice, people tend to lose more, as we also cut out unhelpful processed foods such as artificial sweeteners and sugar, which can disrupt your gut bacteria (microbiome), which in turn can lead to metabolism changes and rampant cravings.

How shall I track my weight and body composition through the three months?

I recommend you weigh yourself at the beginning of this plan and measure your waist (see Chapter 1 for explanation about how to do this correctly).

Use the same set of scales, at the same time of day – preferably naked, when you first get up in the morning. Remember that your weight is influenced by your menstrual cycle (if you are a woman), water retention, if you've had a stool movement recently, exercise and how hydrated you are. Weighing on home scales, even digital, is a very rough measure.

How often should you weigh yourself? The less often the better, in my opinion. I've worked with so many people who use the scales to beat themselves up. The 10-Hour Diet is a gentle, gradual, kind way to lose weight, and a whole lifestyle change. Weight loss can be variable from person to person, and accelerates and wanes at different parts of the three months, according to each individual.

I prefer waist measuring – fortnightly at the most. It's kinder and probably a more accurate assessment of progress, and the area of the body it's most advantageous to lose weight in terms of health (the fat around the organs in your body).

And if you want to see how your muscle mass is progressing (from all that exercise you're doing pre-breakfast!), take a few pictures on your phone privately for yourself, to compare month by month.

If I have to eat late socially, for work, or a celebratory event, what are my options for getting back on track with timings the next day?

Life happens, so be kind to yourself! Count 14 hours forward from your last calorie in the evening and open your eating window later the next day. For example, if you finish the last sip of wine at 10pm, then start your calorie intake 14 hours later, at around noon the next day. Then try to finish eating that day between 6pm and 8pm latest. Basically, you'll be eating in a 6- to 8-hour slot that day, and can get back into a 10-hour rhythm the next day.

You can probably reach your weight-loss and health goals during the three-month period if you end up going off-piste once a fortnight.

What tips are there for riding through late-evening hunger if I experience it in the early days?

You could make your last meal of the day protein-rich (aim for around 20g of protein at this stage). This can help blunt hunger appearing later in the evening, as protein can take a good 4–5 hours to break down in the stomach. You won't need 20g of protein at your evening meal throughout the three months, but I have learnt from my clients' experiences that it is important for extra satiation in the early stages as your hunger hormones rebalance. When this happens, usually after a week or so of 14-hour overnight fasts, you generally feel full up quicker and get hungry slower.

Here are some examples of meals from the recipes given earlier that would help do the trick:

Beans on toast with Worcestershire sauce and cheddar cheese
9g of protein from a 200g portion of baked beans
16g of protein from a 65g portion of grated cheddar cheese
TOTAL – 25g of protein

Sardines on toast with roasted red peppers
24g of protein from a 100g tin of sardines
TOTAL – 24g of protein

Harissa potato with halloumi and green olives
22g of protein from 4 slices of halloumi (100g, or about half a block)
TOTAL – 22g of protein

I don't go into great detail in the recipe section of this book on exact portion sizes – you will be the best judge of that. The tables in Chapter 6 are so you can visualise foods that may be more filling than others and choose accordingly. The reason I tread with such caution around portion sizes and weights is that, in my clinical experience, weighing and measuring food can be a slippery slope. It can become stressful and could trigger what is called ARFID (Avoidant Restrictive Food Intake Disorder).

We are all so individually different in size and nutritional needs, so the best judge of how much food or protein you need is you. 20g of protein is just a rough guideline and may be not quite enough for a 6ft-tall man who regularly goes to the gym, compared with a 5ft-tall woman who leads a sedentary lifestyle.

I invite you to really enjoy food and listen to when you are full and what suits your personal situation and needs. Do make sure that in the early days there is some tasty protein on your plate in your last meal of the day, though, as it may help you forget the fridge later.

For more help, look at Chapter 4 again – go over your top ten supports and the top six non-food treats you wrote down to use as you are getting used to evenings without snacking.

Can I chew gum during the 14-hour fast?

Most gums contain either sugar of some description (so not advisable during your fast) or artificial sweeteners (e.g. aspartame, sucralose, saccharine). Artificial, zero-calorie sweeteners are controversial in the science world. There are fears they may trick the brain into thinking it has had sugar and trigger the production of insulin in some people, leading to fat storage. Some have been shown to disrupt the microbiome (another organ which has control over metabolism) in mice studies. In my opinion we need to know a lot more before including them in our diet at any time of day.

Can I have stevia in my coffee or tea during the 14-hour fast?

Although the zero-calorie sweetener stevia comes from natural plants, it is also controversial, the fear being it could trick the brain into thinking it has had sugar and therefore may lead to fat storage. We need to watch what research shows us about this one in the next few years. Until then, avoid it during your 14-hour fast.

Is it okay to have nut milks in coffee and tea during the fast, as there are so few calories in them?

Nut milks, even if only a few calories, are probably best avoided, as we don't know if they will sabotage your fast and, therefore, the results. In the TRE studies where tea and coffee were allowed, they were taken black. In some studies, the subjects were only allowed water or their prescription medications during the fasting period.

I've noticed that black tea, and some herbal teas, contain one calorie per tea bag when I checked on the pack or on calorie-counting apps. So am I breaking my fast if I have those during my 14-hour fast?

Black tea, which is listed on some calorie-counting apps as containing one calorie, has been used successfully in TRE trials, so I'm happy to use it in the 10-Hour Diet during the fasting period. I've used green tea, white tea (which both contain less caffeine than black), ginger teas, fennel teas, mint teas and chamomile teas successfully with clients too. I'm more wary about including fruit teas during the fasting period. Some contain one calorie per portion, but others contain up to 100! Conclusion: choose teas containing one calorie or less.

Should I eat breakfast?

This is entirely up to you. If you enjoy breakfast and feel hungry in the morning, then enjoy breakfast. If you are someone who doesn't feel hungry naturally until late morning, you might find having two meals a day a better option for you. There are no set rules on this.

Will I still get all the benefits if I just have a few scraps of food in the evening or between meals – e.g. one mouthful of children's leftovers?

Maybe not – so try to fill up at main meals. Throw the children's leftovers in the bin, squirt washing-up over the plates, give them to the dog, put them in the compost bin, brush your teeth – whatever helps you avoid them! I know it can be annoying seeing food go to waste, but we often eat scraps and leftovers because we've been conditioned to avoid waste, rather than because we need food or are actually hungry. Many of us are eating more food than we need to please other people – e.g., the cook or host. You could try taking smaller portions or asking for smaller portions when out and about. You may find you eat more appropriate amounts for your needs and avoid food waste too.

Is it better to do a 16-hour fast as the default, rather than 14, and do you get more benefits the longer you fast each day?

I have tried 16-hour fasting with clients, and it can be effective, but in my experience, and according to some research, longer fasting doesn't seem to be necessarily more effective. The reason researchers are focusing heavily nowadays on 14-hour fasting is because it is simpler to do, feels gentler on the body, is easier to incorporate into life in the long term and yields great results. (See box on p.128–9 for tips on 16-hour fasting.)

Is it okay to snack?

If you are someone having two meals a day, and need a snack in between, then plan and legitimise it. If you are someone having three meals in your 10-hour slot, you may find you don't get particularly hungry and find you don't need a snack. Fill up at main meals, and listen to your hunger cues to decide.

Why isn't time-restricted eating suitable for people with a history of eating disorders?

For those with a history of eating disorders, for example, anorexia, bulimia, or avoidant restrictive food intake disorder (ARFID), there can be an urge to try to push fasting longer and harder – beyond the 14-hour fasting window – which can lead to physical and mental ill health. There is a fine line with fasting between engaging in it healthily and pushing it so far that you become unwell, nutritionally depleted, and engaged in unhealthy thought patterns.

Do you have any tips for engaging in this diet as a night-shift worker?

We know from research that night workers are at high risk of metabolic syndrome – a cluster of obesity, heart disease and type 2 diabetes (described in chapter 1). Working and eating at night, when we are designed to be sleeping, disrupts our hormones and fat-storage mechanisms. For example, we know from studies that more fighfighters die from heart attacks than from fighting fires.

So, if you are in the shift-work world, what could you do to protect yourself? Theoretically, the way to do this would be to eat during the daytime and fast at night even when you are working nights.

For example, you have breakfast when you come off your shift at 8am; sleep for seven hours; have a light lunch around 3pm, then a substantial supper including protein to keep you going a long time, finishing around 6pm. This would mean eating in a 10-hour daytime window.

On days off, try to follow the same eating pattern – breakfast 9am, lunch around 3pm, then high tea finishing by 6pm – as this could help keep your hormones more balanced. Getting 7-plus hours sleep would also be important to help with weight loss.

I know from friends who are ambulance workers, security guards, doctors and care workers that this eating schedule would be challenging. All you can do is what you can and try to keep the times of eating stable, avoiding grazing if at all possible.

Can you get the benefits of the 10-Hour Diet without losing weight? I want to participate in it to try to bring down my blood pressure.

If you don't want to lose weight, or want to limit the amount you lose, I suggest you do this diet for fewer than five weeks and eat more than you usually do in your 10-hour eating window. There isn't a huge amount of research to guide us. In a 2018 study of pre-diabetic men, subjects were fed very large portions between 6.30am and 8.30am (breakfast), at around 10am (lunch), and finished dinner between 1pm–3pm, for five weeks. The men's blood pressure came down and their diabetic markers improved without losing weight.

It's not clear exactly how they managed not to lose weight – maybe they were being fed much more than they normally ate to make up for the very long fasts. They were certainly eating very hearty meals, according to details. Eating earlier in the day is thought to be influential in correcting blood pressure and diabetes markers.

If I already have low blood pressure, will this diet make it go even lower (which I don't want)?

In my experience, fasting helps lower blood pressure when the starting position is at unhealthy high levels. With people whose blood pressure is already in a healthy range, it appears to stay in the healthy range with fasting. This may be because when the body is in a balanced position (called homeostasis), it works to stay there. It is only when a system has become out of balance that it tries to get it back into balance – which is where fasting may help with blood pressure.

Cases of confusion

Sometimes people come to see me in my clinic after they have been trying time-restricted eating on their own for some time.

They have often heard about TRE from blogs, podcasts and/or social media. There is lots of information out there about overnight fasting of different lengths – 12 hours, 14 hours and 16 hours are all popular. Another form of intermittent fasting is 'One Meal a Day', which involves a 23-hour fast!

In Chapter 2 of this book you can read about many of the

different mechanisms in the body that get switched on after 12 hours without food, so you can see why so many different forms of overnight fasting are becoming of interest.

However, sometimes people don't see any results – from weight loss to improved digestive symptoms – even though they have been trying to do long overnight fasting for weeks.

Here are three common actions I've seen by people who thought they were fasting, which may have been sabotaging their attempts to improve their health by way of TRE:

1. Eating mints or chewing gum that contain sugar during the fasting period.
2. Having artificial sweeteners in coffee in the morning (both coffee and artificial sweeteners are laxatives, so if you are using TRE to try to clear up chronic diarrhoea, these are not a good idea).
3. Having almond milk in coffee.

Usually just pushing these items from the fasting period into the 10-hour eating timeslot, and switching the coffee for a black or green tea, makes the fast work properly and they start to lose weight and/or have a normally-formed stool each day.

PUSHING FASTING TOO FAR

I have worked with people who have been delighted to see the pounds falling off and their digestive symptoms improving after fasting. Before working with the 10-Hour Diet, some of my clients tried eating in an 8-hour window and fasting for 16. I generally only suggested this to people who were non-breakfast eaters – the type of people who only feel hungry late morning and say they feel nauseous if they try to eat food soon after getting up.

In the first few weeks, digestive symptoms improved and they lost lots of weight. However, trying to eat in an 8-hour window long term proved difficult for many, and in some cases led to exhaustion and no further weight loss happening. For others, digestive symptoms got worse again. This is why I believe there is a delicate balance with fasting and a sweet spot where it can be done healthily. Here are some examples of what I have seen happen and some of the traps to avoid.

- Trying to push breakfast back later and later, or forgetting to eat, so you end up opening the eating window at 2pm, then counting 8 hours forward and finishing dinner at 10pm. We know from research that successful outcomes from TRE generally happen when participants finish eating before 8pm (preferably 2–3 hours before you go to bed).
- People becoming exhausted after many months of very long fasts (e.g. 16+). I wonder if this is because the eating window is so short (8 hours) that there aren't enough feeding opportunities for some people to get a wide range of nutrition to cover B vitamins,

iron, B12 and folate requirement levels. Or perhaps it's because there are sometimes outside-life stressors, leading to poor sleep (which we know can make fasting potentially dangerous), a halt to any weight loss and an extra strain on the heart. We would need some long-running randomised control trials to get more answers on all this.

- Meanwhile, for some people, 16-hour fasts suit them fine and become a default pattern which works successfully long term. My question is, can younger people's bodies cope with and benefit from longer fasting better than older ones'? Again, we don't have the research to answer this question yet.

CHAPTER EIGHT

Lean for Life: Habits for Long-term Maintenance

You've followed the 10-Hour Diet for three months, lost weight, and now would like to maintain your new weight and metabolic health, from lower blood pressure and better insulin control to better heart markers.

How do you do that?

1. In animal studies, weight and metabolic health was kept stable by practising time-restricted eating five out of seven days a week.

   Could you see yourself doing this? It may be as simple as eating in a 10-hour timeslot, finishing eating between 6pm and 8pm, on the weekdays and being more flexible on weekends. Could you fit your eating into a 12-hour slot instead of 10 at weekends to help maintenance?

2. Human studies have indicated that people find time-restricted eating easy to implement longer term and it can become an engrained habit they find easy. Many are still practising it between 4 and 12 months after the study they had participated in had finished. If you have set new mealtimes in your household, could you keep them going easily? If so, go for it.

Other tips for keeping healthy using time-restricted eating longer term:

1. To maintain lean muscle, make sure you eat enough protein each day. You can check what is the correct minimum amount of protein you need daily with this calculation (mentioned also on page 107).

   Your weight in kilos ____ multiplied by 0.75g = ____
   (Source: Food Standards Agency.)

   Refer to the list of protein foods on pages 108–110 for more guidance on how to fulfil your quota.

   When some people change from eating three meals a day to two a day, sometimes their protein intake goes down, which could affect the amount of muscle they have. For instance, if you used to eat eggs for breakfast, then started cutting out breakfast long term, this could affect your muscle mass, so you would need to bump up your protein intake at the remaining two meals to stay strong. The raw material for making muscle is food containing protein. As we age, part of the ageing process involves our lean muscle mass gradually reducing, so if you are middle-aged or beyond, this is particularly important to keep an eye on if you want to keep lean. If you are vegan or vegetarian, you'll also want to make sure you are getting sufficient protein. A rough guide would be 20g of protein at each main meal. Obviously, this changes depending on your size, but is a simple rule of thumb.

2. Remember that exercise is important for muscle mass (and strong bones) as we age, too. You can maintain and build lean muscle by eating protein and adding some kind of weight-bearing exercise to your routine. This doesn't have to be some major expedition to a formal gym; simply do a set number of press ups, a few downward-dog yoga postures or some quick sets with hand weights at home before you open your eating window. Tagging an activity onto another daily ritual, such as brushing your teeth or waiting for the kettle to boil for your first tea of the day, can be an effective way of building a new movement activity into your routine and remembering to do it. Warm up with a few star jumps or running on the spot

for a minute or two before you start, and find something you enjoy. After all, you are much more likely to keep it going if you like doing it.

A case of editing a 16-hour eating slot down to 10 to help a skin condition

This female had a chronic inflammatory skin condition, and we introduced eating in a 10-hour time slot over three months to help.

When we started working together, the client's food diary was full of nutritious food (as you can see from the example below), so at first it was hard to understand why the inflammation of the skin was bothersome and why the client experienced itching after eating some foods.

A typical day went as follows:

5.45am *Toast, banana, coffee with oat milk*
9am *Coconut water, a cup of coffee*
9.15am *Nut bar*
10am *Biscuit*
1pm *Salad, chicken, pasta, olives, oat biscuits*
3pm *Ginger tea and 2 dates*
8pm *Jacket potato, guacamole, goat's cheese, Parma ham, beetroot*
10pm *Glass of kefir*

As you can see, her eating was spread over almost 16 hours a day (just like the people in the Salk Institute studies we learned about in Chapter 1).

We worked together and reduced the eating window initially to 12 hours a day, and then to 10 hours a day. This was done by waiting until she got to work after 9am before having any food or drink, and making sure supper ended around 7.30pm, with no further snacks afterwards. So, eating was reduced from almost 16 hours a day to around 10.

We also took out alcohol (which was usually just social) and added a wider range of fruit and vegetables to her diet. They contain plant chemicals and fibre, which are food for gut bacteria and make it flourish, which helps reduce inflammation in the body.

This client also stopped snacking and made sure she had three hearty meals per day instead. She was drinking just herbal teas in between meals.

I'm sharing this case with you to show you that tweaking the diet, or slightly upgrading it, as well as having a 14-hour fast, can be worth the effort if you have capacity to combine both.

Here is a snapshot of three days of her new routine of eating. You'll see she has upped her plant intake through lentils and beans, nuts and seeds, and now eats a wider range of vegetables, fruits, herbs and spices. I have indicated where the eating slot starts and finishes, so you can see the window clearly.

Day 1:

6am (wake up):	Mint tea and glass of water
9am (get to work):	Mint tea

Eating slot opens

9.30am (breakfast):	2 x boiled eggs Banana Coffee with oat milk Coconut water
1pm (lunch):	Homemade chickpea salad with leftover roast chicken (would include ingredients such as tinned chickpeas, cucumber, tomatoes, pumpkin seeds, mint, rocket, grated carrot, lemon and olive oil, salt and pepper) Small handful of nuts such as walnuts 2 squares of 85% dark chocolate
7pm (dinner):	Quick and easy homemade dahl made with red lentils, onion, garam masala, turmeric, garlic, chilli, red pepper, spinach, ginger, coriander and lime Stewed apple, flaxseed, cinnamon, goat's milk yogurt Glass of homemade kefir

Eating slot closes at 7.30pm

8.30pm–9:30pm	1 or 2 cups of herbal tea

Day 2:

6.30am (wake up):	Mint tea and glass of water
9am (get to work):	Mint tea

Eating slot opens

9.30am (breakfast):	2 x boiled eggs Cut-up apple and a small pot of peanut butter Coffee with oat milk Coconut water
1pm (lunch):	Salad box from a local deli (mix of healthy salads such as beetroot, lentils, chilli and green-cabbage salad) Small handful of mixed nuts and seeds 2 x squares of 85% dark chocolate Herbal tea
7pm (dinner):	Spiced aubergine with black rice and green salad Glass of homemade kefir

Eating slot closes at 7.30pm

8.30pm–9:30pm	1 or 2 cups of herbal tea

Day 3:

6.30am (wake up):	Mint tea and glass of water
9am (get to work):	Mint tea
Eating slot opens	
9.30am (breakfast):	Porridge with full-fat milk, coconut flakes, flaxseeds, chia seeds, small teaspoon of peanut butter, banana or apple, sunflower seeds Coffee with oat milk Coconut water
1pm (lunch):	2 slices of seeded bread with avocado, sliced tomato and salad leaves A handful of blueberries 2 x squares of 85% dark chocolate Herbal tea
7pm (dinner):	Roast chicken, roast veggies (such as butternut squash, peppers, carrots, red onion) and broccoli Raspberries, goat's milk yogurt, flaxseeds
Eating slot closes at 7.30pm	
8.30pm–9:30pm	1 or 2 cups of herbal tea

As described in Chapter 2, overnight fasting can help reduce inflammation in the body, and shaving down the eating window by more than five hours made a big difference to her symptoms. As I said before, this client was eating healthily before, so the changes to diet were tweaks rather than a complete refurbishment. After three months, her inflamed skin had calmed down significantly.

A case of dropping milk in the morning tea, bringing supper forward and introducing exercise

This woman was eating from the moment she woke up in the morning (cup of tea with milk and a biscuit in bed) until she went to bed and was worried about eating certain vegetables because of her irritable bowel syndrome (IBS).

We worked together for four months using the 10-Hour Diet combined with walking 10,000 steps a day and an exercise class two times a week, and she went from 101kg to 87kg, so a loss of 14kg (more than 2 stone, or 30 pounds). Her IBS and depression symptoms improved, too.

CHAPTER NINE

Conclusion

I hope this book has inspired you to use the timings of when you eat – and don't eat – to improve your health and weight for the long term. Gentle, kind, 10-hour time-restricted eating has helped so many people I have worked with, from reducing weight, balancing blood sugar and improving heart health to more effective digestion and fewer inflammatory issues. I now use it most of the time to keep myself well, too.

To be clear, most people don't wake up one morning and go from all-day grazing to eating two or three regular meals in a 10-hour timeslot each day, followed by a 14-hour fast starting 2–3 hours before bed. It has taken us a few decades of long working hours, stressful commuting, late evening cooking and eating, and 24-hour food availability to get where we are today, eating late at night when we weren't designed to eat. Many people practise and learn to master their new eating timings before a new pattern becomes embedded. If you start with a few hiccups along the way, you will learn from each new day and gradually work up to the new timings that will suit your body and commitments better. Once you have some practice under your belt, keep going until it becomes the new default position. Take your friends and family with you on the journey if you can – they will benefit too. For targeted weight loss or to tackle heart and blood sugar balance issues, you may decide to practise this pattern closely for three months initially. Then, to keep the benefits coming, you could practise the 10-hour pattern on weekdays, eating in a 12-hour slot at weekends.

I'm not a fan of the word 'diet', as in my mind it has short-term connotations. We have used it for this book as it is shorthand for 'eating lifestyle'. As a woman in today's society I have been exposed to many different diets that have come and gone in popularity. I like to think of the word 'diet' in the context of this book as a 'style' of eating that can become part of everyday life for the long term. Remember, until the 1960s and 1970s, many of us were still eating this way. By making just a few tweaks – pushing breakfast a little later and supper a bit earlier – we can all reap the benefits. I'm pleased to see that ongoing research into time-restricted eating is settling on the 10-hour slot as the best combination for the costs involved. As I've outlined in this book, the gentle 10-hour eating pattern should also enable you to include sufficient protein in your diet to maintain your muscle mass and develop a lean body, if that is what you are looking to do.

Most importantly, food is one of the greatest pleasures in life. It nourishes us, fuels us and socialises us with other people. Some of my happiest times in life have been shared around a table of weekend lunch food with people I love. Maybe we will go back to making more of our breakfasts and lunches (and get into high teas again!), now we know how much better it is for us to eat our highest-calorie meal of the day in the daytime. This, really, is why I have written *The 10-Hour Diet*: so that we can all enjoy eating – just at the optimum times of day, so that we can receive the best health benefits from it for the long term.

CHAPTER TEN

Journaling

In this section I'm sharing two templates with you that I have designed to help you to embed two new habits: eating in a 10-hour time slot (front loading your diet earlier in the day if weight loss if your main goal) and widening the range of plants you are eating each week.

The 10-hour training template helps you to monitor sleep, movement and hydration, as well as seeing the opening and closing times of your eating window for one week, and the number of hours the eating window totals. This isn't a competition – it's simply to help you keep a record of your implementation and see where you need to tweak timings to get the best benefits.

The Diversity Challenge worksheet plant-count is an optional extra to do when you have mastered your timings. I find in my clinic that widening the plant count can be an additional support to health and easy if you have the capacity. It can also be fun – they say variety really is the spice of life.

Monday

Date:

How I slept and for how long:

My pre-breakfast movement:

Hydration during my 14-hour fast:

Time my 10-Hour Diet started:

Time my 10-Hour Diet finished:

Total number of hours eating:

Tuesday

Date:

How I slept and for how long:

My pre-breakfast movement:

Hydration during my 14-hour fast:

Time my 10-Hour Diet started:

Time my 10-Hour Diet finished:

Total number of hours eating:

Wednesday

Date:

How I slept and for how long:

My pre-breakfast movement:

Hydration during my 14-hour fast:

Time my 10-Hour Diet started:

Time my 10-Hour Diet finished:

Total number of hours eating:

Thursday

Date:

How I slept and for how long:

My pre-breakfast movement:

Hydration during my 14-hour fast:

Time my 10-Hour Diet started:

Time my 10-Hour Diet finished:

Total number of hours eating:

Friday

Date:

How I slept and for how long:

My pre-breakfast movement:

Hydration during my 14-hour fast:

Time my 10-Hour Diet started:

Time my 10-Hour Diet finished:

Total number of hours eating:

Saturday

Date:

How I slept and for how long:

My pre-breakfast movement:

Hydration during my 14-hour fast:

Time my 10-Hour Diet started:

Time my 10-Hour Diet finished:

Total number of hours eating:

Sunday

Date:

How I slept and for how long:

My pre-breakfast movement:

Hydration during my 14-hour fast:

Time my 10-Hour Diet started:

Time my 10-Hour Diet finished:

Total number of hours eating:

Monday

Date:

How I slept and for how long:

My pre-breakfast movement:

Hydration during my 14-hour fast:

Time my 10-Hour Diet started:

Time my 10-Hour Diet finished:

Total number of hours eating:

Tuesday

Date:

How I slept and for how long:

My pre-breakfast movement:

Hydration during my 14-hour fast:

Time my 10-Hour Diet started:

Time my 10-Hour Diet finished:

Total number of hours eating:

Wednesday

Date:

How I slept and for how long:

My pre-breakfast movement:

Hydration during my 14-hour fast:

Time my 10-Hour Diet started:

Time my 10-Hour Diet finished:

Total number of hours eating:

Thursday

Date:

How I slept and for how long:

My pre-breakfast movement:

Hydration during my 14-hour fast:

Time my 10-Hour Diet started:

Time my 10-Hour Diet finished:

Total number of hours eating:

Friday

Date:

How I slept and for how long:

My pre-breakfast movement:

Hydration during my 14-hour fast:

Time my 10-Hour Diet started:

Time my 10-Hour Diet finished:

Total number of hours eating:

Saturday

Date:

How I slept and for how long:

My pre-breakfast movement:

Hydration during my 14-hour fast:

Time my 10-Hour Diet started:

Time my 10-Hour Diet finished:

Total number of hours eating:

Sunday

Date:

How I slept and for how long:

My pre-breakfast movement:

Hydration during my 14-hour fast:

Time my 10-Hour Diet started:

Time my 10-Hour Diet finished:

Total number of hours eating:

The Diversity Challenge

Write down each different vegetable, herb, fruit, nut, seed, spice, pulse and bean you eat this week. Try to aim for at least 30 different types – but some people even get up to as many as 60 or so, hence there is room in the box below for you to aim high. We now know that eating more than 30 different types of plants each week is important for a healthy microbiome, and a healthy microbiome influences for the better our weight, immune system, mood and digestive health. You can note down one type eaten just once during the whole week. So for instance if you have a green apple, that is noted just one time. If you then have a red apple, that can be noted once, as it is a different type of apple with different plant chemicals in the colours to the green one. The same idea with onions: if you have a spring onion today, have a red one tomorrow, and a white one the next day, so you can note down three different types and feed your gut bacteria lots of different types of plant chemicals and fibre. Good luck!

Date of week started:

1	2	3	4	5
11	12	13	14	15
21	22	23	24	25
31	32	33	34	35
41	42	43	44	45
51	52	53	54	55

6	7	8	9	10
16	17	18	19	20
26	27	28	29	30
36	37	38	39	40
46	47	48	49	50
56	57	58	59	60

Date of week started:

1	2	3	4	5
11	12	13	14	15
21	22	23	24	25
31	32	33	34	35
41	42	43	44	45
51	52	53	54	55

6	7	8	9	10
16	17	18	19	20
26	27	28	29	30
36	37	38	39	40
46	47	48	49	50
56	57	58	59	60

This is where I sign off and hand over to you. I'm excited about the future, our future, and how we can all get healthier, simply by eating earlier as nature intended.

Jeannette Hyde,
BSc (Hons) Nutritional Therapy, mBANT, CNHC

References

Author's note

Almost a third of those surveyed (1.6 million) had gained weight since March 2020 https://covid.joinzoe.com/post/lockdown-weight-gain

Ammar et al. 'Effects of COVID-19 home confinement on eating behaviour and physical activity: results of the ECLB-COVID19 international online survey'. *Nutrients (2020).* https://doi.org/10.3390/nu12061583

Chapter 1: The Simple Science of Eating in a 10-Hour Time Slot Each Day

Hatori et al., 'Time-restricted feeding without reducing caloric intake prevents metabolic diseases in mice fed a high-fat diet', *Cell Metabolism,* Vol. 15 (2012): 848–860.

Chaix, A., Zarrinpar, A., Miu, P., Panda, S., 'Time-restricted feeding is a preventative and therapeutic intervention against diverse nutritional challenges', *Cell Metabolism* (2014). doi: 10.1016/j.cmet.2014.11.001

Zarrinpar, A., Chaix, A., Yooseph, S., Panda, S., 'Diet and feeding pattern affect the diurnal dynamics of the gut microbiome', *Cell Metabolism* (2014). doi: 10.1016/j.cmet.2014.11.008

Gill, S., and Panda, S., 'A smartphone app reveals erratic diurnal eating patterns in humans that can be modulated for health benefits', *Cell Metabolism* (2015). doi: 10.1016/j.cmet.2015.09.005

NHS obesity figures: https://digital.nhs.uk/data-and-information/publications/statistical/statistics-on-obesity-physical-activity-and-diet/england-2020/part-3-adult-obesity-copy

Overweight and obese figures in the US: https://www.cdc.gov/nchs/fastats/obesity-overweight.htm

Sutton, E., et al., 'Early time-restricted feeding improves insulin sensitivity, blood pressure, and oxidative stress even without weight loss in men with prediabetes', *Cell Metabolism* (2018). doi: 10.1016/j.cmet.2018.04.010

Wilkinson et al., 'Ten-hour time-restricted eating reduces weight, blood pressure, and atherogenic lipids in patients with metabolic syndrome', *Cell Metabolism* (2020). doi: 10.1016/j.cmet.2019.11.004

Chow et al., 'Time-restricted eating effects on body composition and metabolic measures in humans with overweight: a feasibility study', *Obesity (2020)*. https://doi.org/10.1002/oby.22756

Ha and Song. 'Associations of meal timing and frequency with obesity and metabolic syndrome among Korean adults', *Nutrients (2019)*. doi: 10.3390/nu11102437

Cienfuegos et al., 'Effects of 4-and 6-h time-restricted feeding on weight and cardiometabolic health: a randomized controlled trial in adults with obesity', *Cell Metabolism* (2020). doi: 10.1016/j.cmet.2020.06.018

Hyde, J., First edition, *The Gut Makeover,* Quercus Books (London: 2015)

Martens et al., 'Short-term time-restricted feeding is safe and feasible in non-obese healthy midlife and older adults', *Geroscience* (2020). doi: 10.1007/s11357-020-00156-6

Parr et al., 'A time to eat and a time to exercise', *Exercise and Sport Sciences Reviews (2020).* doi: 10.1249/JES.0000000000000207

Aoyama and Shibata, 'Time-of-day dependent physiological responses to meal and exercise. Review.', *Frontiers in Nutrition (2020).* doi: 10.3389/fnut.2020.00018

Smith, R., et al., 'Metabolic flexibility as an adaptation to energy resources and requirements in health and disease', *Endocrine Reviews* (2018). doi: 10.1210/er.2017-00211: 10.1210/er.2017-00211

Anton, S., et al., 'Flipping the metabolic switch: understanding and applying health benefits of fasting', *Obesity* (2018). doi: 10.1002/oby.22065

Zarrinpar, A., Chaix, A., Panda, S., 'Daily eating patterns and their impact on health and disease', *Trends Endocrinol Metab (2015).* doi: 10.1016/j.tem.2015.11.007

Saklayan, M., 'The global epidemic of metabolic syndrome', *Hypertension and Obesity* (2018). doi: 10.1007/s11906-018-0812-z

Chapter 2: The Power of the 10-Hour Diet

Anton, S., et al., 'Flipping the metabolic switch: understanding and applying health benefits of fasting', *Obesity* (2018). doi: 10.1002/oby.22065

Paoli et al., 'Review: The influence of meal frequency and timing on health in humans: the role of fasting. *Nutrients (2019)*. doi: 10.3390/nu11040719

McHill et al., 'Later circadian timing of food intake is associated with increased body fat', *American Journal of Clinical Nutrition* (2017). doi: 10.3945/ajcn.117.161588

Chaix, A., Zarrinpar, A., Miu, P., Panda, S., 'Time-restricted feeding is a preventative and therapeutic intervention against diverse nutritional challenges', *Cell Metabolism* (2014). doi: 10.1016/j.cmet.2014.11.001

Zouhal et al., 'Exercise training and fasting. Current insights', *Journal of Sports Medicine (2020)*. doi: 10.2147/OAJSM.S224919

Edinburgh et al., 'Skipping breakfast before exercise creates a more negative 24-hour energy balance. A randomised controlled trial in healthy physically active young men', *Journal of Nutrition (2019)*. doi: 10.1093/jn/nxz018

Chung, K., and Chung, H., 'Review: The effects of calorie restriction on autophagy. Role of aging intervention', *Nutrients (2019)*. doi:10.3390/nu11122923

Sutton, E., et al., 'Early time-restricted feeding improves insulin sensitivity, blood pressure, and oxidative stress even without weight loss in men with prediabetes', *Cell Metabolism* (2018). doi: 10.1016/j.cmet.2018.04.010

Tinsley and Horne. 'Intermittent fasting and cardiovascular

disease: current evidence and unresolved questions', *Future Cardiology (2018)*. doi: 10.2217/fca-2017-0038

Mattson, M., et al., 'Intermittent metabolic switching, neuroplasticity and brain health', *Nat. Rev. Neurosci.* (2018). doi: 10.1038/nrn.2017.156.

Baik, S., et al. 'Intermittent fasting increases adult hippocampal neurogenesis', *Brain and Behaviour* (2019). doi: 10.1002/brb3.1444

Kahleova et al., 'Eating two larger meals a day (breakfast and lunch) is more effective than six smaller meals in a reduced-energy regimen for patients with type 2 diabetes: a randomised crossover study', *Diabetologia (2014)*. doi: 10.1007/s00125-014-3253-5

Guo, Y., et al., 'Intermittent fasting improves cardiometabolic risk factors and alters gut microbiota in metabolic syndrome patients', *The Journal of Clinical Endocrinology & Metabolism* (2020). doi: 10.1210/clinem/dgaa644

Regmi and Heilbronn. 'Time-restricted eating: benefits, mechanisms, and challenges in translation', *iScience (2020)*. https://doi.org/10.1016/j.isci.2020.101161

Chapter 3: Changing Behaviour

McHill et al., 'Later circadian timing of food intake is associated with increased body fat', *American Journal of Clinical Nutrition* (2017).

Neuhouser et al., 'Associations of number of daily eating

occasions with type 2 diabetes risk in the Women's Health Initiative Dietary Modification Trial', *Current Developments in Nutrition* (2020). doi: 10.1093/cdn/nzaa126

Chapter 4: Getting Started

Ikonte, C. et al., 'Micronutrient inadequacy in short sleep: NHANES 2005-2016', *Nutrients (2019)*. doi:10.3390/nu11102335

Chapter 5: How to Practise the 10-Hour Diet

William, M. and Rollnick, S., 'Motivational interviewing' (2020). Guildford Press.

Okauchiet al., 'Timing of food intake is more potent than habitual voluntary exercise to prevent diet-induced obesity in mice', *Chronobiology International (2018)*. doi: 10.1080/07420528.2018.1516672

Parr et al., 'A time to eat and a time to exercise. *Exercise and Sport Sciences Reviews (2020)*. doi: 10.1249/JES.0000000000000207

Wirth et al., 'The role of protein intake and its timing on body composition and muscle function in healthy adults: a systematic review and meta-analysis of randomised controlled trials', *The Journal of Nutrition (2020)*. https://doi.org/10.1093/jn/nxaa049

To join the Zoe project, co-founded by Professor Tim Spector, see website: https://joinzoe.com

Guo, Y., et al., 'Intermittent fasting improves cardiometabolic risk factors and alters gut microbiota in metabolic syndrome patients', *The Journal of Clinical Endocrinology & Metabolism* (2020). doi: 10.1210/clinem/dgaa644

Minich, D., 'A review of the science of colourful, plant-based food and practical strategies for "eating the rainbow"', *Journal of Nutrition and Metabolism (2019).* https://doi.org/10.1155/2019/2125070

Pietrocola et al., 'Coffee induces autophagy in vivo', *Cell Cycle* (2014). doi: 10.4161/cc.28929

Ruiz-Ojeda, F., 'Effects of sweeteners on the gut microbiota: a review of experimental studies and clinical trials', *Advances in Nutrition* (2019). doi: 10.1093/advances/nmy037

Higgins 'A randomized controlled trial contrasting the effects of 4 low-calorie sweeteners and sucrose on body weight in adults with overweight or obesity', Am. J. Clin. Nutr (2019). doi: 10.1093/ajcn/nqy381

Borges 'Artificially sweetened beverages and the response to the global obesity crisis', *PLOs Med.* (2017). doi: 10.1371/journal.pmed.1002195

Wang 'Non-nutritive sweeteners possess a bacteriostatic effect and alter gut microbiota in mice', *PLOs Med* (2018) https://doi.org/10.1371/journal.pone.0199080

Suez, J., et al., 'Artificial sweeteners induce glucose intolerance by altering the gut microbiota', *Nature (2014).* doi:10.1038/nautre13793.

Chapter 6: Real Fast Food

Food Standards Agency, 11th edition, *Manual of Nutrition*, The Stationery Office, (Norwich: 2008)

For more recipes using Aleppo pepper see: Ottolenghi, Y. and Belfrage, I. *Flavour*, Ebury Press (London: 2020).

You can check the protein content of many foods at https://nutritiondata.self.com

Chapter 7: Frequently Asked Questions

Waldman, H. et al., 'Time-restricted feeding for the prevention of cardiometabolic diseases in high-stress occupations: a mechanistic review', *Nutrition Reviews* (2019). doi: 10.1093/nutrit/nuz090

Sutton, E., et al., 'Early time-restricted feeding improves insulin sensitivity, blood pressure, and oxidative stress even without weight loss in men with prediabetes', *Cell Metabolism* (2018). doi: 10.1016/j.cmet.2018.04.010

Lowe et al. Effects of time-restricted eating on weight loss and other metabolic parameters in women and men with overweight and obesity. The TREAT RCT. *JAMA Internal Medicine* (2020). doi:10.1001/jamainternmed.2020.4153

Chapter 8: Lean for Life: Habits for Long-term Maintenance

Olsen, M. K. et al, 'Time-restricted feeding on weekdays restricts weight gain: A study using rat models of high-fat diet-induced obesity', *Physiology & Behavior* (2017). https://doi.org/10.1016/j.physbeh.2017.02.032

Chapter 9: Conclusion

Lee, S. A. et al, 'Determinants of adherence in time-restricted feeding in older adults: lessons from a pilot study', *Nutrients* (2020). doi: 10.3390/nu12030874

Chaix, A. et al., 'Time-restricted feeding is a preventative and therapeutic intervention against diverse nutritional challenges', *Cell Metabolism* (2014). doi: 10.1016/j.cmet.2014.11.001

Chapter 10: Journaling

Rollnick, S. et al., *Motivational Interviewing in Health Care: Helping Patients Change Behavior,* Guilford Press (New York: 2008).

Acknowledgements

Massive gratitude to my agent Claire Paterson Conrad for your vision and encouragement. Thank you to Dr Sarah Jordan, for bringing Claire and I together, and to Jane Haynes, for generously connecting Sarah and I.

Thank you Holly Harris and Kaiya Shang, the publishers with passion, and Sophia Akhtar, Genevieve Barratt and Jessica Barratt of Simon & Schuster for all your support. A book takes a village and I feel blessed to be part of this particular village.

This book is the accumulation of my work in the field with hundreds of people. Thank you all. I learn so much and grow with each session, workshop or retreat. This learning is put together with research from all over the world to make practical sense. Special mention must go to trailblazer Dr Satchin Panda and his team from the Salk Institute who have produced some of the most exciting and relevant research in nutrition during the past century. I hope this book will help bridge the gap from lab to dining table for many people.

Thank you to psychiatrist colleagues Dr Judith Mohring

and Dr James Kustow, and psychotherapist Max Cohen and all at The Integrated Practice, Harley Street, for your keen interest in nutrition and lifestyle medicine as well as your kindness and support.

Dr Dave Chatoor of University College Hospital London – thank you for all your guidance, inspiration and help.

Miguel Toribio-Mateas, thank you for the long chats and taking the edge off the loneliness of writing.

Finally, gratitude for and to my children Max and Hanna (who are now taller and wiser than I am) and Markus for all your love and belief in me.

About the Author

Jeannette Hyde is a leading UK-based Nutritional Therapist (BSc Hons Nutritional Therapy, mBANT, CNHC) and author of trailblazing gut-health bestseller *The Gut Makeover.* She has used time-restricted eating with hundreds of people from all over the world in her virtual clinic and private practice on Harley Street, her group health workshops and retreats in Spain. Through this work and following the latest research, she has nailed what are the intricacies needed in practice to make this new form of intermittent fasting work best for the individual you are and get results.

www.jeannettehyde.com
Instagram @jeannettehydenutrition

Index